High Risk Perinatal Home Care Manual

High Risk Perinatal Home Care Manual

Mary Ann Chestnut, RN

President, Citadel MCH, Inc.
Narberth, Pennsylvania

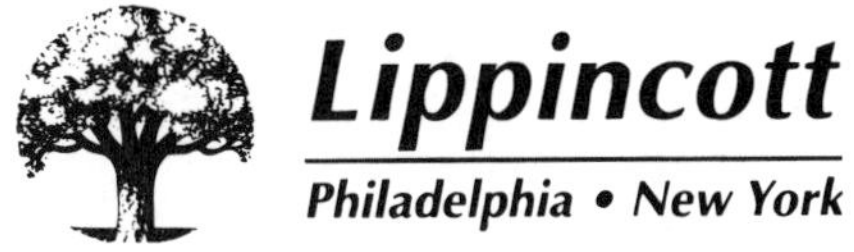

Acquisitions Editor: Jennifer E. Brogan
Coordinating Editorial Assistant: Susan V. Barta
Project Editor: Sandra Cherrey Scheinin
Production Manager: Helen Ewan
Production Coordinator: Patricia McCloskey
Design Coordinator: Kathy Kelley-Luedtke

9 8 7 6 5 4 3 2 1

Library of Congress Cataloging in Publications Data
Chestnut, Mary Ann.
   High risk perinatal home care manual / by Mary Ann Chestnut.
    p. cm.
   Includes bibliographical references and index.
   ISBN 0-397-55478-8
   1. Maternity nursing—Handbooks, manuals, etc. 2. Home nursing—
Handbooks, manuals, etc. 3. Pregnancy—Complications—Nursing—
Handbooks, manuals, etc. I. Title.
RG951.C44 1997
610.73'678—dc21   97-11184
                                                             CIP

This book is dedicated to those whose contributions made this book possible.

*To my husband, Elmer; my parents, Tom and Julia Garvey;
and my children, Kathleen, Tara, Kevin, and Matthew*

To the clients who brought tremendous joy to my life

Thank you

Preface

Today we live in an ever-changing health care environment. During the 1960s and 1970s, perinatal care increasingly turned toward institutionalization. The death in 1963 of President John F. Kennedy's son Patrick at 7 months' gestation provoked a strong movement to examine and find ways to reduce our then 25% infant mortality rate. Perinatal care through this century, but most significantly since the 1960s, has made dramatic advances in the technology needed to improve newborn outcomes. By 1988 the infant mortality rate in the U.S. had been reduced to 10.1%. Although that seems a truly amazing accomplishment, the infant mortality rate has not significantly been reduced since then. In addition, between 1950 and 1952, the U.S. had the seventh lowest infant mortality ranking among 31 countries reporting statistics. By 1988, the U.S. had dropped its ranking to 23rd. In fact, because of the high infant mortality rate among African Americans, the overall infant mortality rate in the U.S. was higher than all other countries except the former Yugoslavia. Recent statistics herald a slight decline in teenage pregnancy, but births to teenagers aged 15 years and younger have increased, and second-time births to teenagers have been on the rise. The total infant mortality rate in the U.S. is also misleading. Neonatal and infant deaths among African American women continue to occur at two to three times the rate of U.S. white infants—most as a result of complications related to low birth weight.

The problem of infant mortality has been studied in great detail by the Institute of Medicine, the National Commission to Prevent Infant Mortality, the Expert Panel convened to determine the Content of Prenatal Care and by at least another 100 large and small organizations. All the studies have reached the same conclusion—adequate access to perinatal care improves pregnancy outcomes. That, however, is not as easily done as said. Only 76% of our mothers currently receive prenatal care.

◾ BARRIERS TO CARE

Multiple reasons exist as to why women do not access prenatal care—inadequate insurance, inadequate number of providers, distance and lack of transportation, and fragmentation of services are just a few. Desire to obtain prenatal care is not enough. We must find ways to improve both access to prenatal care and the quality of care to assure that all women and infants have the best opportunity for the most positive outcome. If prenatal care is to become available to all pregnant women, the population of women receiving inadequate or no prenatal care must be defined and resolved. In addition, all women must have access to comprehensive risk assessment that defines a plan of care specific to their individual needs. In all countries with lower infant mortality rates than the U.S., some degree of home visiting is an integrated component of their prenatal care system. In the Netherlands, 30.9% of pregnant women receive care and give birth at home.[1] In France, women found to be at risk are visited weekly by a sage-femme (a nurse with advanced perinatal training), and they receive a full medical evaluation. Moreover, childbirth classes are provided and necessary laboratory studies are obtained in the at-risk client's home. In 1989 an Expert Panel on the Content of Prenatal Care convened by the U.S. Department of Health and Human Services published *Recommendations for the Content of Prenatal Care*. The panel found evidence of the effectiveness of a regular schedule of home visiting in achieving many of the objectives of prenatal care among women at increased medical and social risk.[2]

The history of maternal-child home care in the U.S. began as early as 1840, with the Manchester and Saltford Ladies Sanitary Reform Associations' Home Visiting Death Reduction Effort. Maternal child home visiting continued to expand until the 1970s, in both public and private agencies, until the technology revolution began to de-emphasize the value of home visiting and focus on institutionally based care. As we prepare to move into the next century with our goals set by the surgeon general for the reduction of infant mortality yet to be realized, we acknowledge that home visiting must be reintegrated as a universally available component of prenatal care as a way to address today's dilemmas.

As of February 1993, the National Association for Home Care identified 13,951 home care organizations in the U.S. The existing provider base in home health offers the opportunity to expand prenatal services programs around the needs and characteristics of the clients, rather than around the habits and traditional orientation of the providers.[3]

The *High Risk Perinatal Home Care Manual* offers a means by which home health providers and practitioners can offer services that are based upon standards of care determined as a result of risk assessment. It also offers a mechanism through which physicians, nurse–midwives, and nurse–practitioners can integrate home health services into the content of their prenatal care programs for those at risk for poor prenatal outcome. Nursing educators will also find this manual helpful in preparing the student for the expanded role of nursing practice within the community.

The first chapter of this manual consists of standards related to the performance of the nurse providing perinatal home care services. These standards will assist the provider in assuring appropriate orientation, training, and job performance.

Chapter two defines the standards for medical and psychosocial standards for risk categories. In order to truly assess client needs, one home visit can provide the picture that is worth a thousand words.

The chapter is divided into three sections. The first section provides directions for the use of a Prenatal Data Collection and Risk Scoring Tool and the Prenatal Universal Home Risk Assessment Tool used in helping to determine the severity of risk and the level of home care services recommended as a result of the risk assessment findings.

Standards determining a level of care assist the home visiting provider in planning a realistic visiting schedule, which is necessary to reach the goals for the individual problems identified in the risk assessment. The psychosocial standards section of the chapter offers an objective means to evaluate the client's needs and reduce the personal judgments we all risk carrying as extra baggage in our work. The physical standards section gives the home visiting provider the clinical norms and the necessary actions to take when deviations are found.

Chapter three offers specific protocols related to the invasive procedures that may be necessary to offer comprehensive home health service to the pregnant client.

Chapter four provides specific protocols for the most common conditions known to cause an at-risk pregnancy. These conditions include premature labor, hypertensive disorders in pregnancy, diabetes, and placenta previa. Additional protocols for frequently used therapies at home for hyperemesis gravidarum for fluids and total parenteral nutrition are also included.

Chapter five offers a perinatal fetal evaluation training program. Providers will find it necessary that all nurses providing perinatal home health services receive training according to defined agency standards to ensure uniform performance and the highest quality of client care. This chapter should be used in the orientation of all nurses to perinatal home care.

Chapter six contains clinical protocols for the delivery of home uterine monitoring services.

Chapter seven presents a three-part childbirth education class that can be offered at home for those clients on bed rest, those with prescribed limitations on physical activity, or those whose geographic region makes access to childbirth education limited. These classes also can be offered in a classroom-type community setting.

Chapter eight offers the provider specific client educational handouts that can be used as teaching tools that can be copied and distributed. These educational tools were developed by Citadel MCH Services and Family Help, Inc., two maternal child specific home health agencies providing services to thousands of clients in the northeastern and southern states of the U.S. The educational handouts have been approved by the clinical advisory committees of these agencies, which consist of maternal-child experts from around the country. The handouts are to be used as general guides; the client should be advised that they do not obviate individual provider instructions.

The Appendices contain actual clinical records that may be used in the provision of care. The Home Health Certification and Plan of Treatment form has been approved by the Health Care Financing Administration of the Department of Health and Human Services for client orders for home health services. The Prenatal Data Collection and Risk Scoring Tool is used to help assess severity of risk and is used to collect data at the time of referral and at the first visit. The Prenatal Universal Home Risk Assessment Tool is used at the first home visit and provides the key to assist in determining the level of care for home visiting frequency. The Perinatal Home Needs Assessment Tool is an addendum form that the nurse may find helpful when collecting more in-depth information, especially related to social issues and problems, as part of the second visit. The Nursing Plan of Care and Progress Record is used for all follow-up visits after the initial home visit. The Discharge Summary form should be completed for all clients discharged from service.

A glossary, bibliography, and list of abbreviations are also included in this manual.

The *High Risk Perinatal Home Care Manual* is the result of more than 10 years of work that I've done in my home health organizations—Family Help and Citadel MCH Services—both licensed, Medicare-certified home health agencies. Family Help additionally received accreditation from the Joint Commission on Accreditation of Health Care Organizations in 1989. I wish to thank the clinical advisory committees of these organizations for helping to establish these standards of care through their input over the years. In addition, I want to acknowledge the contributions of the members of the Pennsylvania Task Force on Maternal Child Home Care (which I organized and chaired from 1991 through 1995) for the voluntary time in developing Recommendations for the Content of Prenatal Care for the state of Pennsylvania. Finally, I wish to acknowledge the contributions of Ellen Craighead, RN, BSN, who worked at Family Help from 1985 through 1990, and whose primary concern was always the clients and their families.

Mary Ann Chestnut, RN

■ REFERENCES

1. Schrivers, A.J.P. & Kodner, L.D. (Eds) (1994). *Health and health care in the Netherlands: A critical self-assessment of Dutch experts in medical and health sciences.* (p. 87). The Ministry of Health, The Netherlands.
2. Public Health Services Department of the U.S. Department of Health and Human Services (1989). *Caring for our future: The content of prenatal care.* (p. 80). Washington, D.C.: Author.
3. The National Commission to Prevent Infant Mortality. (April, 1991). *One stop shopping: The road to healthy mothers and children.* (p. 23). Washington, D.C.: Author.

Acknowledgments

I have been a nurse working in the field of maternal-child health since 1982. Through the years I have had the privilege of working with many individuals who in some way or another have contributed to my knowledge and inspiration to write and publish this manual. I wish to thank and acknowledge the following who have so willingly contributed this support:

The many many staff of Booth Maternity Center, Philadelphia.

The staff at Family Help, Inc: Ellen Craighead, RN, BSN; Marilyn Kerr, RN, BSN; Bonnie Charleston; Anne Ravdin, RN, BSN; Ann Galanter, RN, BS; Joanne Fischer, MSW; Laurie Reardon, RN, BSN; Barbara Tinus, RN, BSN; Gail Pierson, RN, PNP; Barbara Krinsky, RN, BSN; Millie Boettcher, RN, MSN; Patricia Larsen, RN, MSN, CNM; Debbie Westcott, RN, BSN; Judy Woomer, CHHA; and all the other staff who made Family Help a reality.

The staff at Citadel MCH Services: Sonya Newell, RN; Kathleen Whalen, RN; Jacqueline Williams, RN, BSN; Vicki Newell, Carol Hallenback, RN, BSN; Judy Podosky, RN,C; Ann Galanter, RN, BS; and Norma Cintron, RN.

Also a joint acknowledgment must be given to those who served on the The Professional Advisory Committees of Family Help, Inc. (1985–1990) and/or the Professional Advisory Committees of Citadel MCH Services Inc. (1991–1995): the late Paul Branca, MD; Ronald Bolognese, MD; Judy Bernbaum, MD; Evelyn Bouden, MD; Carl Bailey; Jannie L. Blackwell; Roberta Capewell, RN, MSN, PNP; Julia Clarke, RN, CNM, MSN; Jane Eleey, MSW; Jeffrey Gerdes, MD; Page Talbott Gould, PhD; Howard Grant, MD, JD; Robert Holmes, MD; Susan Hutchinson, RNC, MSN; Mark A. Kalchbrenner, DO; Rich Kaplan, MD; June Kinney, PhD; Rose Kinney, RN BSN; Judith McCoyd, ACSW, LSW; Carol L. Natter, PT; Lucille Pema, RN, BSN; Albert Pizzica, DO; Barbara Ritchey, ACSW, LSW; Jeffrey Rothirtan, EdD, PT; Barbara Schraeder, RN, PhD; Robert Stavis, PhD, MD; Patricia Thiebault, RD; Barbara Wesley, MD, MPH; Robert S. Wimmer, MD; Mary Wright, MOT; and Susan Yates, CNM, MSN.

I also want to thank Scott Bucher, RN and My Lo Woodward, RN of the Pennsylvania Department of Health Maternal Child Division and Frank Heron of the U.S. Department of Health and Human Services for their support and assistance throughout the years.

Contents

■ CHAPTER 5

Perinatal and Fetal Evaluation Training Program   105

■ CHAPTER 6

Home Monitoring Program   113

■ CHAPTER 7

Childbirth Education   117

■ CHAPTER 8

Client—Family Teaching Handouts   141

Bibliography   153

High Risk Perinatal Program: Personnel Policies and Procedures and Standards for Nursing Practice

This section provides the basic performance standards for the nurse working in the perinatal home care program. These standards offer guidelines that may be used by agency management and employees to develop expectations of employee practice. They should be used in the orientation of all nursing staff. In addition, the standards provide a mechanism for management staff to measure performance when preparing staff evaluations. These types of policies and procedures are necessary to ensure uniform employee performance, meet federal and state Medicare or licensing requirements, and successfully achieve accreditation by either the National League of Nursing or the Joint Commission for the Accreditation of Healthcare Organizations (JCAHO).

■ PERSONNEL POLICIES AND PROCEDURES AND STANDARD NURSING PRACTICE

The Role of the Professional Nurse Participating in the Family-Centered Maternity Care Program— Perinatal Visit

PURPOSE: To apply uniform quality standards in professional nursing practice related to the perinatal visit within the family-centered maternity care program

RATIONALE: To provide guidelines to the professional employee for expected standards of practice

RESPONSIBLE TO: Director of Nursing

Procedure

1. Receive and record clinical assignment from supervisor.

2. Verify time of scheduled visit with client before arrival.

3. Establish client relationship, using "helping relationship" (Orientation, working, and termination phases (Box 1-1).

4. Review client rights, terms, and conditions of services, including requirements for third-party reimbursement, with client before beginning work.

5. Explain all procedures and rationales to client before performance.

6. Perform assessment of the client's needs (using the Prenatal Data Collection and Risk Scoring Tool and the Prenatal Universal Home Risk Assessment Tool; see Appendices B and C): temperature, pulse, blood pressure, fetal heart tones, uterine activity, Homan's sign, varicosities, edema, vitamins, iron, fluid balance, nutrition, emotional status, and client's knowledge of self-care needs.

Box 1–1: THE HELPING RELATIONSHIP

Orientation Phase: The client will know the nurse by name and accurately describe the roles of the participants in the relationship. The client and nurse will establish an agreement regarding:
- Goals of the relationship
- Location, frequency, and length of contact

Working Phase: The nurse and client work together to meet the client's goals. The client actively participates, cooperating in activities to reach those goals. The client can express his or her feelings and concerns to the nurse.

Termination: The client participates in identifying progress toward or accomplishment of goals. The client verbalizes feelings about the termination of the relationship.

---

7. Provide primary instruction or reinforce individualized prenatal teaching according to the client's condition (rest, activity, diet, elimination, vaginal discharge, sexual activity, maternal activity levels, hygiene, hemorrhoids, exercise, plan for feeding infant).

8. Discuss self-care measures, using concepts of active decision making by client in relation to self-care needs.

9. Discuss methods for preventing problems in the pregnancy (ie, danger signs; see Appendix A).

10. Explain any blood testing or monitoring equipment. Clarify and reinforce physician instructions for follow-up. Verify any questions with caregiver.

11. Evaluate the need for home health aide services or evaluate services if they are being used.

12. Review community resources available to the family (insurance coverage, health clinics, support groups, parenting groups, and so forth).

13. Provide preventive health teaching (breast self-examination, effects of smoking, drugs, diet, caffeine, infant immunizations, need for physical examinations, signs and symptoms of illness in family, and emergency procedures).

14. Review client education materials.

15. For those clients whose caregivers prescribe limitations in activity that prevent attendance at community classes, develop a plan to include childbirth education at home as part of the visit plan.

Perinatal Assessment

POLICY: A prenatal assessment will be performed on all clients referred to the perinatal program.

PURPOSE: To provide nursing assessment for the pregnant woman in the perinatal home visiting program

Procedure

1. The caregiver will ensure that all clients receive information regarding accessing home visiting nurse services.

2. The agency or nurse will contact the client after the referral is received.

3. A visit will be scheduled according to the plan of care.

4. If the nurse is unable to schedule a visit, the nurse will contact the agency regarding the

problem within the first 24 hours after the referral is received. The agency will notify the caregiver and insurer (if required).

5. If the client is a "no-show" when the nurse arrives for the visit, the nurse will contact the agency with a report on the status of the visit and will continue to attempt to see the client, using additional information obtained from the agency, physician, hospital nurse, or insurer.

6. The nurse will obtain a signed consent from the client regarding her home health services.

7. The nurse will perform a physical assessment of the client.

8. The nurse will perform risk assessment and determine potential or existing problems requiring additional home care or caregiver follow-up.

9. The nurse will complete the assessment form for the client, clearly noting the client's insurance number and type, date of birth (DOB), supplemental food program for women, infants, and children (WIC) appointment (if eligible), obstetric caregivers, date and time of follow-up appointment, and all other required information.

10. The nurse will assess client awareness of high risk maternity programs that may be offered by her employer, her insurer, or her county assistance office and recommend follow-up with available programs. The nurse also will provide information regarding county health services for those who are uninsured or eligible for available programs in the community. The nurse will report this information to the agency.

11. The nurse will review emergency numbers and safety measures with the client.

12. The nurse will have the client sign a time log verifying performance of the visit.

13. The nurse will make referrals to other agencies as needed.

14. The nurse will contact the caregiver to discuss findings and develop an ongoing plan for home care or to determine if no further home care is necessary. (In-home health agencies certified by Medicare or accredited by JCAHO, orders for the plan of care must come from a physician.)

15. The nurse will contact the insurer or provide an agency staff member with information to determine whether or not a plan of care for continuing home visits is covered for reimbursement.

16. The nurse will notify the agency when the assessment has been completed and if the client will be referred to the home care program.

17. The nurse will return completed assessments, consent forms, and time logs to the agency.

18. The nurse will contact the client after speaking with caregivers and the insurer to discuss the approved plan of care.

CHAPTER 2

Standards for Risk Categories

The five sections in this chapter are used for two purposes: The first is to collect data indicating whether the client is in a high risk situation. The second is to integrate the data and determine a level of home care based on risks identified and goals to be achieved.

The first section of this chapter provides specific directions for assessing risk and level of care needed. The second section offers a protocol and a tool in which data are collected from the obstetric (OB) care provider, other care providers, and the client herself. The data then are used in a scoring method to determine single or multiple risk factors that in combination place greater stress on the pregnancy. The third section offers the Prenatal Universal Home Risk Assessment tool (also see Appendix C) employed by the nurse on the initial home visit to help determine the appropriate level of care for home visiting services. The level of care is based on identification of factors that assign the client to a preventive, intermediate, or acute level of care. This determination provides an objective means to develop a plan of care and home visiting pattern that can realistically be expected to adequately address both short- and long-term goals. The fourth section of this chapter provides psychosocial standards for the nurse's use when performing the prenatal home risk assessment. These standards provide definitions for the section of the Prenatal Universal Home Risk Assessment tool that is used to determine the level of care. They correspond to the elements on the form to be evaluated (eg, life transitions). The fifth section of this chapter provides standards to be implemented when performing the physical assessment at the initial evaluation visit and at subsequent visits.

DIRECTIONS FOR USE OF THE PRENATAL UNIVERSAL HOME RISK ASSESSMENT TOOL

Assessment

1. The prenatal universal home risk assessment procedure includes
   a. Performing the procedure
   b. The Prenatal Data Collection and Risk Scoring Tool (see Appendix B)
   c. The Prenatal Universal Home Risk Assessment tool
   d. Prenatal Risk Assessment Standards

2. The Prenatal Data Collection and Risk Scoring Tool uses a scoring system based on all previous and current problems that may place the pregnancy in some degree of jeopardy. The scores are determined by affixing a numeric value to historical or existing issues that affect the well-being of the pregnancy. The higher the score, the greater the risk the client experiences in reaching a positive outcome. This tool helps to identify those women who would potentially benefit from a home health program and also provides a mechanism to assure uniform data collection.

3. The Prenatal Universal Home Risk Assessment tool helps to determine a level of home care service, which assists the nurse to plan and provide effective interventions in a universally standard manner. The plan of care then can be individualized to meet the client's needs. The tool uses both the psychosocial and the physical standards that are included in this chapter. In performing the physical assessment of the pregnant woman, nurses can turn to the standards to determine normal limits, deviations, and actions. The psychosocial standards were developed as a tool to promote objective assessment. The psychosocial risk assessment within the tool itself contains eight categories: life transitions, emotional status, substance abuse/risk-taking behaviors, parenting issues, educational/cultural factors, economic/resource needs, maternal medical/nutritional factors, and environmental factors. For each of these categories, corresponding guidelines are presented in the Standards for Psychosocial Risk Categories section of this chapter.

4. Referrals for initial visits can be made by the client's physician, nurse-midwife, nurse, social worker, the client herself, an outreach worker, or another significant person involved in the client's care.

5. The agency, provider, and insurers will make all attempts to determine if client has or has had previous home care services in this pregnancy to avoid duplication of services.

6. Clients will be advised of client rights in advance, in compliance with Medicare, state licensure laws, and Joint Commission on Accreditation of Health Organizations (JCAHO) standards.

7. All plans of care will be supervised by a physician in compliance with Medicare, state licensure laws, and JCAHO standards.

8. It is recommended that all pregnant women, but especially those at the poverty level, be afforded access to prenatal universal home risk assessment to determine risk factors not obvious at the prenatal office visit.

9. Clients will receive a prenatal universal home risk assessment. Women identified with the following admission criteria will be admitted to home care:
    a. Lack of health insurance coverage*
    b. Previous low birth weight, preterm birth, or intrauterine growth retardation
    c. Inadequate prenatal care in this pregnancy
    d. Current/recent drug abuse
    e. Education below 9th grade level
    f. Adolescent age 18 years or younger with first birth
    g. Age 20 years or younger with a second or additional birth
    h. Premature labor
    i. Diabetes
    j. Hypertension
    k. Intrauterine growth–retarded fetus
    l. Inadequate prepregnancy weight and prenatal gain
    m. Other medical or social problems determined by physician that justify providing prenatal universal home risk assessment and ongoing access to home care.

10. Problems identified will be reported to OB caregiver. A plan of care is developed for clients with the above admission criteria. Clients not meeting admission criteria will have community service plan developed by caregiver, with input from the findings of the prenatal universal home risk assessment.

11. As part of the screening, the nurse will complete both the physical and psychosocial risk assessment to help identify and better qualify and quantify client needs for services in the home and community. The prenatal universal home risk assessment standards should be

Agencies should contact the state or local county assistance to enroll in available provider programs to facilitate Medicaid enrollment, which can retroactively cover visits and promote access to care for the client. Federal, state, and the local Department of Health's Maternal Child Division also may have project funding available.

applied to better assure objective predictability of service use and fewer variations in quality and quantity.

Levels of Care

12. After the initial evaluation, a plan of care is developed. The goals and objectives of the plan are based on the individual client needs found through the screening. In the risk assessment section of the Prenatal Universal Home Risk Assessment tool in Appendix C, the problems have corresponding numbers, indicating a level of care (eg, 1. cultural beliefs; 2. inadequate food; 3. current/recent abuse of drugs). The levels provide guidelines that the agency, caregiver, client, and insurer can use to realistically plan for home care service needs, directing the greatest intensity toward the factors having the greatest risks for poor outcome or preventable hospitalization.

■ INITIAL PLAN GUIDELINES

No addition is needed when scoring the risk assessment section of the Prenatal Universal Home Risk Assessment tool. Clients whose risks are all 1s are a level I, clients with all 2s are a level II, and clients with all 3s are a level III.

Many clients will have combinations of 1s, 2s, and 3s. Combinations are not graded based on the quantities of 1s, 2s, or 3s; even one score in the next level entitles the client to the higher level of care. Therefore, a client with three 1s and two 2s would initially start care in the level II category, rather than level I. The nurse and caregiver may determine that the goals of the client's home care plan can be met with three visits the first week and one visit a week thereafter. A client scoring two 1s and five 2s may have a plan in which it will be necessary to visit three times a week for the first 2 weeks and then wean visits to one to two a week for the next 2 weeks.

The visit plans according to levels of care are only guidelines. They offer a realistic visit pattern, which the nurse can use to plan for adequate intervention and teaching time in which to achieve client health outcome goals in a manner that can be adjusted to fit the individual client's needs.

1. Level I: One to three per month first 30 days, then reevaluated every 30 days throughout pregnancy unless discharged

2. Level II: One to three visits per week, reevaluated every 30 days through pregnancy unless discharged

3. Level III: Four to seven visits per week, reevaluated after the first month and then every 30 days throughout pregnancy unless discharged

Medical History Section

13. This section of the form is intended to document maternal medical or OB history or current conditions that may impact on the outcome of the pregnancy. Some of this informa-

tion comes directly from the client at the first home visit, and some comes from the Prenatal Data Collection and Risk Scoring Tool, which documents information from the client and all other health care providers from whom the nurse may receive current or historical information. The first column of the Prenatal Universal Home Risk Assessment tool lists the various medical conditions to be considered. The second column is used to document whether:

    a. The condition was present previously, but is not a problem at this time, which would be indicated by a *p*.

    b. The condition is present at this time, which would be documented by a *c*.

    c. The condition was present previously and is also present at this time, which would be documented by a *p* and a *c*.

14. The third and fourth columns are used to document who will be providing follow-up care (the OB caregiver, the home care nurse, the social worker, etc.). The fifth column is used to provide specific clarification of the condition noted. Clients are discharged based on goals being met or:

    a. No identified admission criteria justifying home care after initial prenatal screening visit

    b. Admission criteria problem identified and resolved

    c. Goals in established plans of care have been met

    d. Goals cannot be met and reasons justified

◼ HOME CARE RECOMMENDATIONS BY RISK CATEGORY

All pregnant women will receive an initial home visit for physical and psychosocial assessment and determination of level of risk.

Initial Risk-Specific Home Care

1. Increased Risk Level I

   All pregnant women determined to have one or more level I risk factors are eligible for one to three visits per month, dependent on individual need and primary care provider's plan of care. This eligibility lasts for 62 days and is reevaluated every 30 days.

2. Moderate Risk Level II

   All pregnant women determined to have one or more level II risk factors would be eligible for one to three visits per week, dependent on individual need and primary care provider's plan of care. This eligibility lasts for 62 days and is reevaluated every 30 days.

3. Maximal Risk Level III

   All pregnant women determined to have one or more level III risk factors would be eligible for four to seven visits per week, dependent on individual need and primary care provider's plan of care. This eligibility lasts for 62 days and is reevaluated every 30 days.

Ongoing Risk-Specific Home Care

The risk status of each pregnant woman will be reevaluated every 30 days or more frequently if needed. The overall plan will be totally reassessed every 62 days, and, dependent on individual risk level and need, a new physician's plan of care may be developed and implemented.

■ PROTOCOL FOR COLLECTION OF DATA

To decrease morbidity and mortality among infants and mothers, a risk assessment at the beginning of pregnancy is essential. Two basic tools can be used to establish and identify a client at risk:

1. Prenatal Data Collection and Risk Scoring Tool (See Appendix B)

2. Prenatal Universal Home Risk Assessment tool (See Appendix C)

Protocol for Assessing Risk (Using the Prenatal Data Collection and Risk Scoring Tool)

1. Characteristics of client at risk
   a. Maternal age
      1) Younger than age 15 years at conception
      2) Older than age 35 years at conception
   b. Weight
      1) Underweight—100 lbs or less
      2) Overweight—more than 20% over standard weight
   c. Height
      1) Short stature—50 inches or less
   d. Race (genetic problems related to specific races)
      1) African American race—sickle cell anemia
      2) Jewish race—Tay Sachs
   e. Marital status
      1) Single
      2) Separated/divorced
      3) Widowed
   f. Culture (specific practices of a culture that would affect pregnancy)

g. Education and occupation

   1) Less than high school diploma

   2) Other than skilled professional workers

h. Socioeconomic factors

   1) Lack of money for prenatal care

   2) Environment/living conditions

   3) Drug addiction or ingestion

   4) Alcoholism

   5) Smoking

   6) Emotional stress (fear, anger, anxiety/tension, family problems, lack of support, ambivalence, client perceptions such as knowing something is amiss)

2. Previous OB history

a. Previous outcomes of pregnancy

   1) Early fetal loss (two pregnancies terminated before 28 weeks)

   2) Late fetal loss (one or more at 28 weeks or greater)

   3) Live premature babies (two or more under 2500 g)

   4) Early neonatal death (one or more under 7 days old)

   5) Early fetal loss and live premature (one fetal loss under 28 weeks in last two pregnancies plus one live premature baby)

   6) Large infant (greater than 4000 g)

   7) Infants being small for gestational age (SGA)

   8) Stillbirths

   9) Intrauterine fetal demise (IUFD)

   10) Intrauterine growth retardation (IUGR)

      (a) Asymmetric

      (b) Symmetric

   11) Chromosomal anomalies

b. Parity

   1) Multipara (more than four pregnancies)

   2) Primigravida

c. Previous surgical or medical intervention delivery

   1) Cesarean section

   2) Version

   3) Vacuum extraction

   4) Mid to high forceps

   5) Breech extraction

   6) Uterine surgical repair (uterine anomaly)

      7) Infertility surgery

      8) Myomectomy

  d. Previous prenatal occurrences

      1) Premature labor

      2) Diethylstilbestrol (DES) exposure

      3) Incompetent cervix

      4) Premature rupture of membranes (PROM)/chorioamnionitis

      5) Perinatal Infections

         (a) Cytomegalovirus (CMV), toxoplasmosis, group beta streptococcus, herpes, hepatitis, rubella

      6) Habitual abortion

      7) Blood sensitization

         (a) Rh

         (b) Irregular antibodies

      8) Hematologic diseases, abnormalities

         (a) Idiopathic thrombocytopenia purpura

         (b) Sickle cell anemia

         (c) Placenta previa

         (d) Chronic placental abruption

         (e) Vaginal bleeding of unknown cause

      9) Acquired immune deficiency syndrome (AIDS)

     10) Pregnancy-induced hypertension (PIH); preeclampsia, eclampsia

     11) Gestational diabetes

     12) Renal disease/pyelonephritis/urinary tract infections

     13) Multiple gestation

3. Medical, surgical history

  a. Hypertension

  b. Renal disease

  c. Diabetes

  d. Cancer within last 5 years

  e. Thyroid disease, endocrine disorder

  f. Hereditary disorders

  g. Cardiovascular disease

  h. Respiratory disease

  i. Hematologic disease/disorder

  j. Collagen disease

  k. Psychiatric disorder

l. Mental retardation

m. Infertility

n. Infectious diseases

o. Neuromuscular disorders

■ STANDARDS FOR PSYCHOSOCIAL RISK CATEGORIES

Purpose

The purpose of standards is to provide the health professional with a screening tool to use in interviewing clients and identifying referral possibilities. The primary use of the form is in risk assessing and referring pregnant women and infants for risk-appropriate services.

The asterisk (*) denotes priority referrals that demonstrate the highest level of risk, indicated as level 3 or maximal level of care on the Prenatal Universal Home Risk Assessment tool, however, in all cases, professional judgment must be used. Any factor or combination of factors could indicate a need for a referral if the professional performing the assessment thinks that the client would benefit. Interdisciplinary cooperation should be assured!

Note: The Prenatal Universal Home Risk Assessment Tool is used for this section and the next section—Standards for Perinatal Physical Risk Assessment.

Life Transitions

Life events that result in the possibility of changes in lifestyle, perceptions, behaviors, belief systems

1. Denial or rejection regarding pregnancy: Denial is defined on a cognitive and emotional level as not acknowledging or accepting the pregnancy. Rejection is defined as a strong negative emotional or behavioral response to being pregnant

2. History of being or current or recent incest or rape victim: Any evidence of sexual abuse or assault (ie, incest, rape)

3. History of infant or child chronic disability: Any diagnosed chronic physical or mental disability in another child

4. History of fetal death or other infant or pregnancy loss: Any loss that has occurred either prenatally or during the infant's first year of life

5. Adoption or termination considered: Client or family seriously considering adoption or termination of pregnancy

6. Suspected domestic violence: Suspected battering of significant other or child or both. Possible law enforcement involved

The Prenatal Data Collection and Risk Scoring Tool
Antepartum Risk Scoring Index

Patient's Name ____

Address ____

Phone number _______________________   Insurance company _______________________

OB care provider _______________________   Phone number _______________________

Gestational date _______________________   Today's date _______________________

A score of 10 or more on this index indicates a client is at high risk.
However, in assessing your future course of action with each client, look at absolute scores instead of just the designation of low or high risk. For example, the diabetic client with no other problems rates 10 points and therefore is considered at high risk. However, the obese client (5) who has a drinking problem (5) and is a heavy smoker (5) scores 15 points; she may be at still greater risk.

Scoring Value	Condition	Actual Score of Client
Anatomical Abnormalities		
10	Uterine malformation	( )
10	Incompetent cervix	( )
10	Abnormal fetal position	( )
10	Hydramnios	( )
5	Clinically small pelvis	( )
10	Multiple pregnancy	( )
10	Vaginal spotting	( )
Miscellaneous (this pregnancy)		
5	Age 15	( )
5	Age 35	( )
5	Weight 100 lbs.	( )
5	Weight 200 lbs.	( )
1	Mild anemia, 9.0–10.9 hemoglobin	( )
5	Severe anemia, 9.0 hemoglobin	( )
10	Sickle cell disease or trait	( )
5	Rh sensitized, first time	( )
5	Positive serology	( )
5	Positive PPD	( )
3	Viral disease	( )
3	Flu syndrome	( )
3	Vaginitis	( )
5	Abnormal cervical cytology	( )
10	Pulmonary dysfunction	( )
10	Post-term (over 42 wk)	( )
10	Intrauterine growth retardation	( )
5	Emotional problems	( )
5	Smoking	( )
5	Alcohol abuse	( )
5	Excessive drug use, nonnarcotic	( )
10	Narcotic use	( )
10	No-care client (no previous medical care until late in pregnancy)	( )

(continued)

Scoring Value	Condition	Actual Score of Client
Cardiovascular Disorders		
10	Class I heart disease	( )
10	Severe heart disease, classes (II–IV)	( )
10	Chronic hypertension	( )
3	History of preeclampsia	( )
5	History of eclampsia	( )
5	Mild preeclampsia	( )
10	Moderate–severe preeclampsia	( )
Renal Disorders		
5	History of GU infection (including acute cystitis)	( )
10	Acute pyelonephritis	( )
10	Moderate–severe renal disease	( )
Metabolic Disorders		
3	Family history of diabetes	( )
5	Diabetes (Type II, III, IV)	( )
10	Diabetes (Type I)	( )
5	Thyroid disease	( )
3	Previous endocrine ablation	( )
History		
3	Therapeutic abortion	( )
5	Habitual abortion	( )
10	Previous stillbirth	( )
10	Previous low birth weight infant	( )
10	Previous neonatal death	( )
5	Previous infant >10 lbs	( )
3	Previous cesarean section	( )
1	Rh neg., nonsensitized	( )
10	Rh neg., sensitized	( )
5	Multiparity >5	( )
5	Epilepsy	( )
5	Previous fetal anomalies	( )
3	Drug allergy	( )

Emotional Status

Client's or significant other's identifiable affect (demeanor, emotional tones), mental status (intellectual functions, use of defenses, orientation to place, person, time), and emotional status (emotional control, emotional appropriateness)

1. History of mental illness or mental health treatment or hospitalization: Diagnosis of mental illness, which may have included outpatient treatment

2. Unresolved grief or significant loss: Inability to reach acceptance in dealing with significant losses, which may include death of significant other, loss of job or home, financial security, divorce, loss of relationship with significant other

3. Suicidal ideation: Serious suicidal tendencies as indicated by verbal threats, extreme depressed states, history of previous suicide attempts, or an actual suicide plan

4. Feels isolated, alone or has inadequate support system: Expression of extreme loneliness. Client may have family members or significant others present but they provide none or only minimal emotional or financial support. Client may not have any support.

5. Questionable coping: Difficulties in adjusting to and accepting social relationships, life opportunities, activities of daily life, self-concept

6. History of postpartum depression: Evidence of a debilitating postpartum depression after a previous pregnancy (eg, inability to take care of personal needs, inability to bond with or care for the infant, potential abuse or neglect of self or infant).

7. Evidence of low self-esteem: Verbal or nonverbal expression of low self-esteem, evidenced by lack of eye contact, downgrading oneself, disheveled appearance, withdrawn, negative self-concept

Substance Abuse or Risk-Taking Behavior

The nurse will assess for ongoing use or abuse of substances and evidence of risky behavior (eg, multiple sex partners, no birth control method, tobacco use, behavioral problems in general)

*1. Current or recent abuse of alcohol or drugs: Ongoing or use within past year of alcohol or drugs as it impacts on the developing fetus, individual, and family. Includes clients with no recent abuse, but still living with other substance abusers

*2. Current or recent abuse of street drugs: Ongoing or use within past year of illicit drugs (eg, heroin, marijuana, cocaine, barbiturates, amphetamines) or a referral from a drug abuse program. History of use or continuing abuse as it impacts on fetus, individual, and family. Includes clients with no recent abuse, but still living with other substance abusers

*3. Current use or recent abuse of prescribed medication: Ongoing or history of use of prescribed medication as it impacts on the developing fetus, individual, and family. Includes clients with no recent abuse, but still living with other substance abusers

4. Law enforcement involvement: Law enforcement involvement with regard to how it impacts on the client's ability to access care or to care for the child.

5. Sexual risk-taking behaviors: Includes but is not limited to multiple sex partners and unsafe sex practices. Includes those who live in crack houses

6. Tobacco use or secondhand smoke exposure: Ongoing use of tobacco (ie, cigarettes, chewing tobacco, snuff) by the client and its impact on the developing fetus or the risk of secondhand smoke exposure to infants/children

Parenting Issues (Observed or Expressed)

Parenting issues are defined as the client's perception of themselves in the role of a parent or the actual behaviors that are observed or expressed by the client.

1. Teen or inexperienced parents: The particular developmental stage of the parents and how it impacts on their ability to parent or nurture the child. Examples: a child raising a child or inexperienced parent exhibiting lack of confidence and fears regarding ability to meet the needs of the child

2. Development issues (child or family expectations): Lack of knowledge or poor understanding of what is age-appropriate for developing child. Expectations are inappropriate, which may lead to punitive responses, such as expecting an 18-month-old to toilet train, and then punishing if child continues to have "accidents."

3. Discipline issues: Discipline methods are often culturally learned behaviors. Problems occur when discipline is not appropriate to the child's development stage. Example: disciplining a crying 3-month-old because the infant is perceived as being bad and deliberately crying to upset the parents

4. Relationship issues (bonding or nurturing): Poor eye contact, cold, not able to cuddle with infant (which can lead to failure to thrive).

5. Child abuse or neglect history, now resolved: History of placement of another child because of abuse or neglect, currently resolved

6. Child abuse or neglect, current: Uncertainty regarding the possibility of abuse or neglect, and anyone with current Child Protective Services involvement. The staff person who directly observes such behavior is required by law to report it. Ensure interdisciplinary involvement and follow-up.

7. Three or more children younger than 6 years of age: Possibility of increased stress related to care of multiple children younger than 6 years with few parental support or social outlets.

Educational or Cultural Factors

These are factors that are associated with higher than average infant mortality or morbidity or that might impede a client's ability to follow instructions, meet expectations, or adhere to a recommended plan of care. Referrals might enhance the likelihood of appropriate use of services.

1. Low literacy or limited intellectual ability: Evidence of inability or difficulty in reading basic instructions. Documentation of low or borderline intellectual capabilities

2. Language barriers: Unable to communicate basic information in English; also includes hearing and speech impairments

3. Cognitive deficits: Documented or perceived deficits in the ability to process information

4. Educational level 12th grade or below: Failure to complete school beyond grade 12

5. Educational level 10th grade or below: Failure to complete school beyond grade 10

*6. Educational level 9th grade or below: Failure to complete school beyond grade 9

7. Culture or beliefs: Identify and acknowledge cultural factors and beliefs that may impact health attitudes and behaviors such as religious beliefs and practices, health values, attitudes toward getting and receiving health care, and current behaviors and lifestyle. These factors vary among communities and individuals, and providers should be prepared to identify and respond to the needs of the populations that they serve.

Economic or Resource Needs

These factors could be appropriately handled through case management or, if more than one factor presents significant stress, through psychosocial intervention.

1. Insufficient income or no income to meet basic needs

2. No transportation: Unable to secure adequate transportation to meet instrumental activities of daily life. This may include a client's inability to plan or to take responsibility for required decision making.

3. Inadequate food: Difficulty in obtaining food to meet basic nutritional needs. May include lack of resources to purchase food or lack of knowledge about available resources

4. Legal needs: Need for assistance from the legal system (eg, child support, divorce, domestic violence). May include lack of resources to secure legal aide or empowerment to effectively access legal resources available

5. Chronic difficulty accessing system: Persistent inability to access multiple agencies to assist with resources, impairing the ability to meet the most basic needs

6. Child care problems: Problems securing adequate acceptable child care such that the ability to gain employment or to access medical care is difficult or of low priority

7. Medicaid problems: No existing permanent medical coverage for term of pregnancy

Maternal Medical or Nutritional Factors

1. Abnormal physical findings this assessment: Any abnormal findings as noted on page 1 of the Prenatal Data Collection and Risk Scoring Tool

2. Problems with chosen family planning method: Unable to successfully use existing family planning methods. May be medical or emotional reasons

3. Short interconceptual period: Interconceptual period of less than 1 year between this conception and the preceding delivery

4. Grand multigravida: Pregnant more than seven times

5. Anemia: Hemoglobin <10.8 g/dl. If client does not know, ask if folic acid has been prescribed

6. Chronic disease: Medically diagnosed and documented chronic disease (eg, diabetes, hypertension, renal disease, cardiovascular disease, liver disease, tuberculosis, sickle cell disease or trait, cancer, seizure disorder, and so forth)

*7. Human immune deficiency virus (HIV) positive/AIDS: Any client or significant others with medically diagnosed and documented HIV or who has tested positive for AIDS virus

8. Problem initiating breastfeeding: Any failed attempt at breastfeeding

9. Pica: The eating of substances not ordinarily considered edible or to have nutritive value, such as dirt, clay, or laundry starch

10. Anorexia, bulimia or fad diets: Suspected or medically diagnosed and documented case of anorexia or bulimia or eating disorders; follower of fad diets (eg, grapefruit diet, diet pills, and so forth)

*11. Inadequate prenatal care: Fewer than four prenatal visits, for any reason

*12. Previous preterm birth, low birth weight, intrauterine growth retardation, or preeclampsia: Any previous pregnancy that was complicated by preterm birth, low birth weight, IUGR, or preeclampsia

Environmental Factors

1. Housing problems include any of the following:
   a. Inadequate living space or accommodations to meet the number of occupants in the household such that a health or safety hazard potentially exists
   b. Conditions that are substandard such that clear safety hazards exists (Poor sanitation, ventilation, or heating; electrical hazards; vermin infestation)
   c. Movement from one house, apartment, or shelter to another without stable home base or network of support systems. This could include the migrant population.
   d. Without housing or totally reliant on community support for shelter or living on the streets

2. Utilities: Lack of electricity, heat, phone, or air conditioning when they are basic necessities

3. Water or Sewer: Lack of water or sewer facilities

4. Refrigeration: Lack of refrigeration

5. High risk or unsafe neighborhood: Neighborhood is an area of high crime or otherwise known to be unsafe for its residents. This would include a known drug area.

6. Inadequate preparation for infant: Lack of preparation for meeting the basic needs of a newborn in the home (no crib, car seat, clothing, or formula)

◼ STANDARDS FOR PERINATAL PHYSICAL RISK ASSESSMENT

Temperature

1. Standards within normal limits (WNL): Oral temperature between 97 F and 100.3 F.

2. Deviations: Oral temperature above 100.4 F.

3. Evaluation of deviation: Temperature up to 100.4 F not unusual if unaccompanied by other symptoms. If temperature persists for 48 hours, it is abnormal. Check for other symptoms such as leaking of fluid from the vagina, calf or leg pain, undue pain or discomfort, burning on urination.

4. Action: If temperature is between 99 F and 100.4 F, check for premature rupture of membranes, urinary tract infection, or other systemic infection. Call caregiver from client's home and relate findings, if suspected infection or rupture of membranes. If infection not suspected, mother should be instructed in signs and symptoms of infection and to retake temperature every 4 hours. She should report signs and symptoms (see Appendix A: Danger Signs) of infection—persistent temperature elevation over 24 hours or a rise in temperature to above 100.4 F—to her physician.

Pulse

1. Standards WNL: Pulse rate between 50 and 100 beats per minute (BPM). Occasional heart palpitations because of increased workload on heart.

2. Deviations: Pulse <50 or >100 BPM.

3. Evaluation of deviation: Pulse rates >90 BPM could indicate either infection, hidden bleeding, or severe anemia. Check to see if other signs, such as hypotension, vaginal fluid or bleeding, diaphoresis, or pale skin color, also have deviated from norm. Tocolytic agents used for premature labor may increase heart rate and respiratory rate to above the normal

standard. Assess frequency of palpitations to determine whether they are occasional without incident or persistent and indicative of cardiac irregularity.

4. Action: If pulse rate is >90 BPM and other signs are evident, call physician from client's home immediately and relate findings.

Blood Pressure

1. Standards WNL: Blood pressure remains in accord with previous readings if there were no problems. 90/60 to 140/90 mmHg is a good range. Deviations must be measured against the average blood pressure of individual client. Blood pressure history must be obtained from client.

2. Deviations:
   a. Sustained rise of 30 mmHg or more in systolic blood pressure
   b. Sustained rise of 15 mmHg or more in diastolic blood pressure
   c. A sustained systolic blood pressure of 140 mmHg or more
   d. A sustained diastolic blood pressure of 90 mmHg or more (Journal of Nurse Midwifery, Vol. 39, No. 2, March/April 1994)

3. Evaluation of deviation: The work of the cardiovascular system is increased during pregnancy because of the excess fluid normally acquired in pregnancy. Evaluate to determine if edema and headache are present. Borderline BP of >130/80 mmHg or rising BPs should be monitored more closely. Preeclampsia develops after 20 weeks and is characterized by +1 or greater proteinuria and >1+ nondependent edema. Elevated BP in early pregnancy is related to chronic hypertension. Most women with mild hypertension have fairly uncomplicated pregnancies. Preeclampsia, however, when combined with chronic hypertension, is most associated with severe maternal complications.

4. Action: If the client has an increase in blood pressure along with blurred vision, headache, epigastric pain, or edema, call a physician immediately. If elevated without other symptoms, take blood pressure in both arms. If evident in both arms, have client lie down for 15 minutes and retake. If the client has decreased BP and is asymptomatic, instruct the client to notify the physician if she becomes symptomatic.

Gastrointestinal System

1. Standards WNL: Decreased peristalsis caused by the effect of progesterone on the smooth muscle of the bowel may contribute to constipation and increased flatus. Iron supplements

and changes in diet, activity, and exercise are also contributing factors. The effects of progesterone in relaxing the cardiac sphincter along with decreased gastrointestinal motility and the compression of the stomach by the enlarging uterus contribute to heartburn as a discomfort. Adequate weight gain is 16 to 35 pounds.

2. Deviations:

   a. Nonexistent bowel sounds

   b. Inability to have a bowel movement accompanied by pain, fever, vomiting, suspicion of intestinal obstruction or impaction, frequent watery diarrhea stools that could contribute to dehydration

   c. Poor weight gain or obesity

3. Evaluation of deviation: Auscultate for bowel sounds in client. Obtain a history of client's eating and normal bowel pattern. If client is in any pain, determine if vital signs are within normal limits. Pain in the mid to upper right in back should be evaluated for gallbladder problems. Provide nutritional counseling according to client needs.

4. Action: If bowel sounds are nonexistent, contact caregiver. If bowel sounds are present but client has not moved bowels, the recommendations are exercise, increased roughage in diet, and increased fluids. Instruct client to notify caregiver if no relief from constipation is obtained as a result of these measures or if pain, vomiting, frequent watery stools, or temperature are present. Clients taking iron will have better absorption if it is taken with a large quantity of vitamin C–enriched fluids. Caregiver should be notified if iron continues to cause a problem because another form might be prescribed.

Urinary System

1. Standards WNL: Average output is 1,500 mL per 24-hour period via urinary tract

2. Deviations:

   a. Decreased output of less than 30 mL/hr

   b. Dysuria

   c. Frequent urination with small amounts of urine

   d. Pain with chills and fever

3. Evaluation of deviation: Evaluate client's voiding patterns. Determine whether client has had difficulty voiding and whether caregiver is aware of this. Check client's temperature.

4. Action: Notify caregiver from client's home if signs and symptoms of urinary tract infection or bladder distention are present.

Breasts

1. Standards WNL: Two mammary glands with a wide, pigmented areola. Sometimes a less pigmented area, called the secondary areola, is present. Venous engorgement may be visible, along with striations of the skin. The nipple is erect and deeply pigmented. Some clients may have flat or inverted nipples. Most women experience an increase in breast size during pregnancy as a result of the expanded body fluid volume and growth of glandular and lobular breast components. Nipples and areola may become darker during pregnancy. Toward the end of pregnancy, yellow fluid called colostrum may begin to appear. Nipple stimulation practiced by many women in preparation for breastfeeding should be avoided for those experiencing premature labor. Nipple stimulation causes the release of oxytocin in the brain, stimulating the uterus to contract.

2. Deviations: Presence of any masses in the breasts, discomfort as a result of heaviness and increased size

3. Evaluation of deviation and actions: Immediately notify caregiver of any breast masses found; instruct client to wear supportive bra to promote comfort.

Fundus or Uterus

1. Standard WNL: Abdomen is soft, tender, no masses. After 22 to 24 weeks, the uterus size is measured in centimeters from the symphysis pubis to the top of the fundus; the number of centimeters should equal approximately the number of weeks' gestation, within 2 weeks. Client may complain of Braxton Hicks contractions in the second and third trimesters. These are mild arrhythmic contractions without the presence of labor. Fetal heart tone should be between 120 and 160 beats/min.

2. Deviations: Excessive uterine irritability (contractions), severe pain or tenderness, fundal height consistently more or less than expected, fetal heart tones below 120 or above 160 beats/min

3. Evaluation of deviation: Contact caregiver from home if labor contraction or ruptured membranes suspected before 37 weeks, or whenever there is severe pain or tenderness unrelated to normal labor after 37 weeks. Encourage increased fluids and lying on left side. Contact caregiver immediately if fetal heart tones are not within normal limits.

4. Action: Notify caregiver immediately from client's home if premature labor is suspected, or in the presence of any bleeding suspected to be from the uterus or gush of fluid from the vagina before 37 weeks. Fetal bradycardia could be the result of compression and should be

treated as a true emergency. Fetal tachycardia indicates compromise of the fetus, and the caregiver should be notified immediately.

Perineum

1. Standards WNL: The normal vulva of a pregnant woman will appear increasingly swollen as the pregnancy progresses because of increased fluid volume, impaired venous circulation, and increased venous pressure in the lower extremities. These changes are also caused by the pressure from the enlarging uterus on the pelvis veins contributing to venous stasis. Increased vaginal discharge is normal in pregnancy.

2. Deviations: Vulvar varicosities, hemorrhoids, excessive or green, yellow, foul-smelling, or irritating vaginal discharge

3. Evaluation of deviation: Contributing factors include family tendency, increased weakness of the vascular walls attributable in part to increases in progesterone. Obesity, poor muscle tone, and inactivity also irritate. Constipation associated with pregnancy also contributes to hemorrhoids. Deviations in vaginal discharge may be caused by venereal disease, trichomonas vaginitis, or moniliasis.

4. Action: Notify caregiver from client's home if client is having extreme pain not relieved by normal techniques such as sitz bath and analgesics. Notify physician also of bleeding or severe swelling. Encourage client to cleanse perineal area from front to back and to use good hand-washing technique. Instruct client to maintain diet to reduce constipation, perform Kegel exercises, sitz baths, witch hazel compresses, adequate rest and exercise, to avoid sitting or standing too long in one place, and to not cross legs, and to use support hose and elevate hips and legs when resting.

Extremities

1. Standards WNL: Increasing mobility of sacroiliac, sacrococcygeal, and pelvic joints results from progesterone changes, which contribute to alteration of maternal posture and to back pain. Vascular congestion may occur in pelvic region, contributing to varicose veins in the lower extremities, vulva, or pelvis. In addition, pressure from the gravid uterus may contribute to hemorrhoids, leg cramps, or edema of the lower extremities.

2. Deviations: Pain, tingling, feeling of leg giving out, phlebitis, bleeding hemorrhoids, painful, pitting edema

3. Evaluation of deviation: Evaluate back pain to determine whether pressure on sciatic nerve is interfering with mobility. Evaluate extremities for warm reddened areas that may be indica-

tive of phlebitis. Determine whether pain from hemorrhoids interferes with elimination or whether they are bleeding. Assess whether fatigue or dietary deficiencies in calcium contribute to leg cramps. Assess edema in extremities to assure that it is not associated with hypertensive states.

4. Action: Notify OB care provider for severe back pain that extends down one or both legs. Notify OB care provider for suspected phlebitis not under treatment; reinforce bed rest and fluids. Rule out vaginal bleeding as source and consult OB provider for care of bleeding hemorrhoids. Notify OB care provider of pitting edema in which client's blood pressure is 140/90 mmHg or there has been an increase of 30 mmHg systolic or 15 mmHg diastolic.

Psychological Status

1. Standards WNL: Pregnancy has a strong psychosocial and physiologic impact, which causes the woman to be challenged by the developmental tasks of pregnancy. These can include unusual thoughts and desires related to food, sex, fatigue, mood swings, increased sensitivity, frustration, and vulnerability.

2. Deviations:
    a. Acting out behaviors that place the pregnancy at risk (eg, lack of interest in self-care, risk-taking behaviors, prolonged depression)
    b. Maladjustment to body image changes

3. Evaluation of deviations: Evaluate for signs of depression or dangerous behaviors that risk safety or physiological well-being, such as detachment, disinterest in personal appearance and nutrition, anxiety, anorexia, and exaggerated fatigue. Expresses strange or inappropriate thoughts or feelings, delusions, hallucinations, or hostility toward significant other and medical staff.

4. Action: Consult with physician as to the best plan of action. Emphasize the need for follow-up visitation prenatally and postnatally because client may be at risk for severe postpartum depression or psychoses.

CHAPTER 3

Invasive Procedures

The perinatal home care plan may need to include invasive procedures performed by the nurse. These primarily involve intravenous therapy and venipuncture blood specimens collected for laboratory analysis. Intravenous therapy is used for such conditions as hyperemesis, infection, total parenteral nutrition, and in some cases, hydration in premature labor. Serial blood collection may be required for a variety of reasons, including complete blood count, serum, chemistries, and so forth. The nurse performing these procedures should be experienced in venipuncture or should receive a 3-month formal training program approved by the agency's advisory committee, of which one member will be a certified intravenous (IV) nurse. For nurses inexperienced in IV therapy, one-on-one training with an experienced IV nurse should be required through the entire orientation. The ability to provide IV therapy at home reduces the need for hospitalization, thus keeping the family together. The ability to have blood collected at home as part of the visits reduces the risk of premature labor in clients with physical limitations that require them to reduce the frequency of trips to the laboratory facility.

■ POLICY AND PROCEDURE: PERIPHERAL VENIPUNCTURE TO INSERT A CATHETER

POLICY

The nurse will maintain patency of peripheral line for infusion therapy, as prescribed.

PURPOSE:

To access and maintain peripheral patency for prescribed administration of fluids and medication on a continuous or intermittent basis.

Procedure

1. Equipment needed
   a. Tape
      1) Exception: Nonallergic tape is used on excoriated skin
   b. Intravenous cannula as appropriate
   c. Sharps container
   d. Normal saline
   e. Latex gloves
   f. Heparinized saline concentration
   g. Transparent dressing
   h. Injection cap
   i. Alcohol swabs
   j. Povidone-iodine swabs

2. Frequency
   a. Intravenous site rotation every 3 days or more often as needed for phlebitis, thrombosis, infiltration, infection, or other problems (unless otherwise ordered by obstetric [OB] caregiver)

3. Procedure
   a. Explain procedure to client.
   b. Prepare clean work surface.
   c. Organize supplies needed.
   d. Wash hands (following hand-washing procedure) and put on latex gloves.
   e. Selection of IV cannulas
      1) Butterflies
         (a) 23- and 21-gauge butterflies are most frequently used.
         (b) For difficult venous access, a 27- or 25-gauge butterfly may be used.

   f. Catheters

     1) Size ranges from 14- to 24-gauge catheter.

       (a) Gauge of needle depends on client needs.

     2) Catheters are used over butterflies when:

       (a) Infusing a drug or solution that is very irritating to the vein

       (b) Infusing via pump

  g. Selection of insertion site

     1) Examine all extremities for venous access.

     2) Start examining distally and work proximally toward the client.

     3) Only superficial veins are to be used.

     4) Contraindications of placement

       (a) Infection, osteomyelitis, cellulitis; do not use affected extremity

       (b) Vasospasm secondary to deep lines with discoloration of an extremity; do not use the affected extremity

     5) Preparation of site

       (a) Use a circular motion, cleansing first with alcohol wipes, then wash the area with povidone-iodine swab and allow to dry for 20 seconds.

  h. Insertion of cannula

     1) Apply tourniquet to dilate the vein.

     2) Site may be numbed with 0.1 or 0.2 mL normal saline intradermally, using a 27- or 26-gauge needle (optional).

     3) Hold catheter comfortably and firmly for insertion, and secure the vein below the insertion site with the other hand.

     4) Insert the needle, bevel up, through the skin parallel to the vein, until blood return is achieved. Thread cannula until hub is proximal to the skin surface.

       (a) NOTE: Pre-stick with a 21- or 22-gauge needle for a 22- or 24-gauge catheter to ease insertion may be used (optional).

     5) No more than three attempts may be made by one nurse.

  i. Secure cannula in place with tape.

     1) Do not apply tape too tightly, as pressure sores may occur, especially under the hub of the catheter.

     2) Do not place tape directly over the site.

     3) Apply povidone-iodine ointment to all catheters and transparent dressing over the insertion site.

  j. Remove tourniquet and stylet.

  k. Connect either IV tubing or injection cap (heparin lock) into cannula and secure.

    1) For injection cap (heparin lock), flush with heparin, and check for patency by aspirating for blood return and observe for signs or symptoms of infiltration.

    2) Routine flushing

    3) Minimum flushing of injection cap (heparin lock) is once per a day when not in use.

l. Documentation of insertion site, gauge of catheter, date and time of insertion, nurse's initials, and any complications of the procedure. These should be noted on nursing progress notes.

m. Inform client and parent or caregiver of signs and symptoms of complications and rationale and performance of this procedure as appropriate.

n. Discard all used materials in sharps container.

o. See Table 3-1: Guidelines for Problematic Client Conditions, for treatment of problems.

■ POLICY AND PROCEDURE: PERIPHERAL VENIPUNCTURE—BLOOD DRAW

POLICY   Nurse will properly draw blood with a peripheral venipuncture as per orders

PURPOSE: To obtain a venous blood sample for prescribed laboratory studies to obtain
                          and maintain proper mode of treatment

Procedure

1. Equipment needed
    a. Vacutainer
    b. Tubes
    c. Needles
    d. Tourniquet or rubber band
    e. Alcohol swabs
    f. Povidone-iodine SWABS
    g. Cotton ball or 2 × 2 sterile gauze sponge
    h. 1″ Adhesive bandage
    i. Sharps container
    j. Gloves (latex)

2. Procedure
    a. Explain procedure to client and parent/caregiver.
    b. Assemble all necessary equipment.
    c. Wash hands thoroughly as per procedure and put on latex gloves.
    d. Assess status of upper extremities for venipuncture site. After site has been selected, apply tourniquet or rubber band. Tourniquet or rubber band should be tight enough to trap venous blood but not interfere with arterial flow. If radial pulse cannot be palpated, tourniquet or rubber band is too tight.
    e. Clean area with povidone-iodine swab or alcohol iodine swab; allow to dry.
    f. Prepare collection tube and needle for insert.
    g. Stretch skin below the vein by holding it firmly with thumb so skin is held taut. This will prevent the vein from rolling away from the needle. Make venipuncture with needle bevel up. Enter the skin at approximately a 30-degree angle. Once needle is through the skin, decrease the angle by lowering the needle hub nearly flush with the skin, and continue inserting with a straight, forward motion.
        1) NOTE: Frequently, you will feel sensation of "release" when you enter the vein.

TABLE 3-1
Guidelines for Problematic Client Conditions

Client Condition	Effect on Client	Guidelines
Shock, sepsis, hypotension	Poor perfusion; vasoconstriction; difficult to locate veins	1. Flush fluid through needle. 2. Use different tourniquet tensions or blood pressure cuff techniques. 3. Expect no blood return. 4. Inserter rarely feels needle enter the vein. 5. Soaks may help but are not very effective. 6. Squeeze distally and proximally to site at the same time to pump up the vein.
Increased temperature; febrile	Dilated veins	1. May not get blood return. 2. Usually easier to find veins.
Decreased body temperature due to cold environment, use of cooling mattress, use of multiple swabs with alcohol on babies	Vasoconstriction	1. Apply warm soaks over a large area. 2. Wrap with blanket and wait 30 minutes. 3. Use warmer bed if available. 4. Use different tourniquet tensions or blood pressure cuff techniques. 5. Expect not much blood return.
Fear vasoconstriction	Fight or flight	1. Controlled breath; stick vein when client is exhaling. 2. Have client blow out candles or shout ''Ouch!''
Jaundice or bililights (phototherapy); low platelets	Fragile veins	1. Apply low tourniquet tension. 2. Enter vein slowly and advance gently. 3. Remove tourniquet rapidly.
Malnutrition: Poor skin turgor, poor muscle tone	Large, unstabilized veins	1. Exaggerate skin tension. 2. Insert whole unit in the vein before advancing the catheter.
Flaccidity: Very poor muscle tone, loose skin	Rolling veins not visible or palpable.	1. Rely on anatomy. 2. Exaggerate skin tension. 3. Use of the veins of the feet is usually easier.
Obesity	Veins not visible	1. Digital veins are often visible. 2. Rely on anatomy. a. Press out fluid.
Edema	Veins not visible	1. Test for refill. 2. Insert needle far enough into the vein so that returning fluid will not push the needle out.
Long-term therapy	Damaged veins; many collateral veins	1. Use any guidelines as necessary.

h. Withdraw appropriate amount of blood, changing blood tubes if necessary.

i. Remove tourniquet or rubber band.

j. Remove needle and apply pressure with 2 2 2 sterile gauze sponge to site. After bleeding stops, apply bandage. Discard all used sharps and materials in sharps container.

k. Document the procedure on nursing progress notes.

l. Label the tubes of blood with client's name, date, time, nurse's initials.

m. Notify case manager of where the blood specimen is being processed.

Guide for Blood Tube Collection

1. Blood tubes

   a. Red tube: Nonpreserved, plasma and cells separate; electrolytes, chemistries

   b. Gray tube: Fasting blood sugar, 2-hour postprandial, and random blood sugars

   c. Blue tube: Prothrombin time, partial thromboplastin time

   d. Purple tube: Complete blood cell count, hemoglobin, hematocrit

   e. Green tube: Carbon dioxide content, electrolytes

   f. Navy blue tube: Trace elements

2. Notes

   a. Different tubes have different preservatives.

   b. Preservative-containing tubes should be filled first and gently rotated.

   c. Ideally, tubes should be filled to capacity to have proper mix of blood with preservative.

   d. Verify tube preference with local laboratory, because some laboratories may use different-colored tubes.

   e. Store blood samples in cool, dry place until they can be brought to the appropriate laboratory.

■ POLICY AND PROCEDURE: PERIPHERAL LINE— HEPARIN LOCK APPLICATION

POLICY   Nurse will insert and maintain heparin lock patency as prescribed.

PURPOSE: Maintain an intravenous line with a heparin lock for clients requiring venous access for medication. Allow client freedom of mobility.

Procedure

1. Follow nursing procedure for peripheral venipuncture; assessment of site, insertion of catheter, and taping of site.

2. Flush heparin lock with 0.5 mL to 1 mL heparin flush solution (1 mL normal saline/10 units heparin solution) at time of insertion of heparin lock and after each dose of medication.

3. In giving medication dose, heparin lock is flushed with 0.3 mL normal saline, then medication is administered, followed by 0.3 mL normal saline flush, and then heparin flush (1 mL normal saline/10 units of heparin solution).

4. Assessment of IV site at time of flushing for infiltration, phlebitis and/or leaking

5. Document on Nursing Medication Sheet and Nursing Progress Notes the following information:
   a. Date and time heparin lock was started
   b. Date and time site was changed
   c. Gauge of intravenous needle
   d. Medication administered
   e. Assessment of site

6. Properly discard materials in sharps container.

7. Educate family member (caregiver) about the procedure for applying pressure to site if heparin lock should become dislodged.

■ POLICY AND PROCEDURE: PERIPHERAL INTRAVENOUS COMPLICATIONS

POLICY　　　　　　　Nurse is competent to recognize signs and symptoms of peripheral intravenous therapy complications.

PURPOSE:　　　　　Promote expedient recognition and appropriate intervention for complications of intravenous therapy.

Procedure

1. Phlebitis
   a. Inflammation of the walls of the vein
   b. Cause: Direct injury or trauma to the vein from intravenous injections, indwelling catheters, overuse of a vein, infusion of an irritating solution, use of a large-bore cannula, long-term cannula placement, or extension of an infection into the tissue surrounding the vessel.
   c. Symptoms: Venous distention, edema, local heat, erythema, induration, or pain at the site of cannula placement and along the course of the affected vein
   d. Intervention: Identify and document symptoms, change IV site, apply cold compresses for 24 hours and moist heat thereafter to stimulate circulation and promote absorption. Continue observation for elevated temperature, purulence, pain, erythema, or local heat at identified site. Notify OB caregiver of intervention, and obtain further prescribed orders.

2. Thrombosis
   a. Clot formation in cannula or vessel that occludes flow through the catheter or vessel
   b. Cause: Usually caused by stasis of blood in catheter by client position, neglectful heparinization of catheter
   c. Symptoms: Inability to flush catheter, erythema, inflammation, induration of insertion site
   d. Intervention: Discontinue peripheral intravenous line according to procedure. Notify OB care provider and proceed as prescribed.

3. Infiltration
   a. Accumulation of fluid in tissue surrounding intravenous cannula
   b. Cause: Dislocation of cannula or loss of vessel integrity
   c. Symptoms: Edema, skin blanching, pain, decreased temperature of skin at site, and slowing or cessation of intravenous fluid not associated with mechanical or tubing problems.

    1) NOTE: A blood return may still be present with infiltration.

  d. Intervention: Discontinue infusion and cannula. Apply warm compresses to site of infiltrate to increase fluid absorption. Notify OB care provider and proceed as prescribed.

4. Embolism

  a. Obstruction of blood vessel by a blood clot or a foreign substance

  b. Cause: Most common is dislodging of a thrombus into systemic circulation

  c. Symptoms: Ischemia, hypotension, dyspnea, cyanosis, tachycardia, peripheral numbness, tingling, and loss of consciousness

  d. Intervention: Call OB care provider immediately and initiate emergency procedure, as should be stated in the policies of all providers of this service.

    1) NOTE: If a catheter fragment has entered into the systemic circulation, immediately apply firm pressure (proximal manual tourniquet) to contain the fragment.

5. Infection

  a. Intravenous site that has been invaded by pathogenic organisms, producing deleterious effects locally and systemically

  b. Cause: Poor aseptic technique, contamination of catheter or solution and intrinsic factors (immunosuppression, steroid therapy, or malnutrition)

  c. Symptoms: Fever, chills, tachycardia, erythema inflammation, purulence, pain, localized heat from insertion site

  d. Intervention: Prevent infection by inspecting solution and supplies for contamination. Properly review and perform aseptic technique. Notify OB care provider of signs and symptoms and proceed with prescribed orders.

6. Teaching caregivers and clients

  a. With all of these complications, the caregivers and clients are to be educated regarding the following information:

    1) The condition and definition of the condition

    2) Symptomatology

    3) Proper interventions

    4) All teaching by infusion nurse is documented and reviewed at each visit.

■ POLICY AND PROCEDURE: DISCONTINUATION OF PERIPHERAL INTRAVENOUS CATHETER

POLICY

Nurse will discontinue peripheral intravenous catheter properly when prescribed.

PURPOSE:

To remove an intravenous cannula when intravenous access is no longer prescribed or when site rotation is necessary or when complications exist.

Procedure

1. Put on latex gloves.

2. Place gauze over the site of the cannula insertion and withdraw cannula.

3. Hold gauze in place with slight pressure for 2 to 3 minutes.

4. Check site for continued bleeding.

    a. NOTE: If bleeding continues, apply pressure or pressure dressing.

5. If no bleeding exists, apply bandage or gauze with tape.

6. Discard materials in sharps container.

7. Document on Nursing Progress Notes time, date, and assessment of site after discontinuation.

CHAPTER 4

Specific Protocols for the High Risk Pregnant Woman

This section of the manual offers care providers very specific treatment protocols. These protocols were developed to address the three most common causative conditions that have been linked to poor pregnancy outcome, low birth weight, and intrauterine growth retardation. These conditions include premature labor, hypertension, and diabetes. The protocols have been used with hundreds of clients, producing significantly improved outcomes over those of the overall population with the same risk factors.

Low birth weight is a major determinant of infant mortality in the United States. The risk of mortality increases as birth weight decreases. The goal of any intervention program is to identify those factors known to be associated with low birth weight outcome and eliminate, or at least reduce, those risks. These protocols combined with the assessment tools offer a means to identify those risks and develop a home visiting treatment plan that maintains appropriate levels of care for the home visit. In its 1989 publication "The Content of Prenatal Care," the United States Department of Health and Human Services discusses home visiting. Its Expert Panel, which convened for several years to study this issue, recommends home visiting as an effective means of intervention, especially to those at risk. These standards also offer a tool through which an agency or insurance provider can evaluate the risk characteristics of the population within their service area for planning purposes.

In addition, protocols are offered that address hyperemesis gravidarum, total parenteral nutrition, training the perinatal nurse, home uterine monitoring, and childbirth education. These protocols may be copied and included in each nurse's orientation, acting as a resource and standard of care for the perinatal client. The childbirth education section of the manual offers a resource for the nurse to use in teaching, which also may be copied and given to parents participating in these sessions. A parent section includes other teaching materials for distribution.

■ PERINATAL HOME CARE PROTOCOL FOR PREVENTION OF PREMATURE LABOR

Eligibility

Once the client is identified as high risk on the Prenatal Data Collection and Risk Scoring Tool (see Appendix), arrangements must be made for emergency transportation.

Risk Factors

1. Major risk factors
   a. Previous premature labor
   b. Multiple gestation
   c. Diethylstilbestrol (DES) exposure, associated anomaly
   d. Cone biopsy history
   e. Cerclage
   f. Abdominal surgery in second or third trimester
   g. Polyhydramnios
   h. Uterine anomaly
   i. Irritable uterus
   j. Medical or obstetric problem history
   k. Economical/social maladaptations

2. Minor risk factors
   a. Bleeding after 12 weeks of gestation
   b. One or more previous first trimester abortions
   c. One previous second trimester abortion
   d. Pyelonephritis
   e. More than 10 cigarettes per day

General Nursing and Treatment Orders

1. Referral from obstetric (OB) care provider to high risk home visiting program.

2. OB care provider refers the client's history, antenatal testing, and laboratory values to the agency.

3. The clinical administrator notifies client of referral and explains the prevention program.

4. The clinical administrator assigns a perinatal nurse to complete an initial prenatal evaluation visit.
   a. Prenatal evaluation visit will include

1) Physical and psychological assessment using the Prenatal Universal Home Risk Assessment tool, which, combined with the information obtained from the Prenatal Data Collection and Risk Scoring Tool, will help to determine the appropriate level of care for home visiting patterns and interventions.

2) Complete obstetric, medical, surgical history.

3) Social and economic assessment

   (a) Establishing whether client needs home health aide services or any other community resources (support groups)

4) Education of client and family about premature labor (risk factors, controlling, and prevention)

5) Providing educational material on premature labor

6) Agency nurse will leave the agency number for any problems.

7) A plan of care is established between client, nurse, OB care provider, and insurer.

8) Nurse will provide a schedule of when client's visits will occur.

5. The perinatal nurse will report initial prenatal visit to clinical administrator.

6. The clinical administrator will discuss with referring OB care provider the plan of treatment after the initial prenatal visit, if there are any issues or problems surrounding the plan of treatment.

Nursing Assessment

1. Activity
   a. Limited activity up until 20 to 24 weeks, then possibly bed rest with bathroom privileges, because risk for premature labor increases later in pregnancy.
   b. Lateral side passive exercises
   c. Range-of-motion exercises

2. Diet
   a. Well-balanced meal for pregnant mothers
   b. Increase in fluid hydration

3. Education
   a. Prepare client for premature delivery and caring for a premature infant.
      1) Educational material on premature delivery infants, recommended reading for the mother (eg, *Premature Baby Book,* by Helen Harrison and A. Kositsky, St. Martin's Press, New York, 1983, or *Pregnancy at Bed Rest,* by Susan H. Johnston and Deborah A. Kraut, St. Martin's Press, New York, 1990)
      2) Education of client and family members about premature labor

        (a) What is a contraction?

        (b) What are the causes of premature labor?

    3) Notify OB care provider if having increase in regular contractions.

    4) Educate client on actions and side effects of any tocolytic agents.

    5) If used, evaluate uterine monitoring system twice per day for 1 hour each time. OB care provider should be contacted if there are four contractions per hour.

    6) Provide emotional support.

        (a) Perinatal nurse listens, provides information about client's diagnosis and positive reinforcement.

        (b) Support groups: Establish a phone connection with other clients at home in premature labor as well as other clients who have experienced premature labor with a positive outcome.

  b. Prepare client for childbirth education at 30 weeks' gestation.

  c. Offer information about possible passive range-of-motion exercises by 32 weeks' gestation.

4. Follow-up care

  a. Establish with client that after delivery, follow-up appointment with OB care provider is necessary.

  b. Encourage client to establish a yearly appointment with her OB care provider.

5. Individual Treatment Plan

  a. Level I: Preventive

    1) Nursing visits: Weekly visits; can be decreased to once every other week.

    2) Home health aide: 3 to 5 days per week

  b. Level II: Intermediate

    1) Nursing visits: 2 to 3 times a week for first 2 to 3 weeks, then decreasing to once per week.

    2) Home Health Aide: 3 to 5 days per week.

  c. Level III: Acute

    1) Nursing visits: Daily visits starting day of referral. Weekly reports to OB care provider, or, if there is a problem, more frequently

    2) Home health aide: 5 to 7 days per week. Maintain bed rest; prepare for premature labor, delivery, or possibly premature baby; introduce childbirth education.

▉ PERINATAL HOME CARE PROTOCOL FOR PREMATURE LABOR

Eligibility

1. Identified as being a high risk client

2. History of premature labor

3. Onset of regular uterine contractions without cervical dilatation

4. No tocolytics

5. No placement of cerclage

6. Identified as high risk through use of Prenatal Data Collection and Risk Scoring Tool

Once a client is considered at risk for premature labor, arrangements must be made for emergency transportation. If there is economic hardship, utilities companies also must be notified of a need for water, phone, and heat.

General Nursing and Treatment Orders

1. OB care provider refers client to agency high risk perinatal program.

2. Plan of treatment is established between referring OB care provider, client, nurse, and insurer, if required.

3. The perinatal nurse is assigned to complete an initial prenatal evaluation visit by the clinical administrator. The prenatal evaluation visit includes
   a. Physical and psychological assessment using the Prenatal Universal Home Risk Assessment tool, which, when combined with information obtained from the Prenatal Data Collection and Risk Scoring Tool, will help to determine the appropriate level of care for home visiting patterns and interventions.
   b. Complete obstetric, medical, and surgical history
   c. Social and economic assessment
      1) Establish whether client requires home health aide services or any other community resources (support groups).
   d. Provide for education of client and family about premature labor (risk factors, control, and prevention of premature labor).
   e. Agency nurse will leave the agency number in case of any problems.
   f. A plan of care is established between client, OB care provider, nurse, and insurer.
   g. Nurse will provide a schedule for client visits.

4. If indicated, the home uterine monitoring system will be initiated at 20 weeks' gestation.

a. Perinatal nurse will collaborate with the monitoring system to establish a plan of treatment for the client.

b. Instructions will be given to the client on the operation of the equipment.

　　1) Monitor two times per day for 1 hour each time.

　　2) If contractions increase within 1 hour, lie on left lateral side and increase fluid hydration. Monitor in 1 hour.

　　3) If uterine contractions persist at more than five in 1 hour, notify the OB care provider.

　　4) The client will be directed to the regional perinatal emergency room, or the agency's perinatal nurse will be called to evaluate the situation in person if symptoms do not indicate imminent danger or delivery.

　　5) Perinatal nurse evaluates the presence of five or more contractions. If there is no cervical dilatation, IV hydration may be initiated per OB provider's order.

　　6) Nursing visits by a perinatal nurse at the initiation of the home monitoring system shall occur at least two times the first week; then once per week up until 34 weeks' gestation; finally, once per week or every other week as needed, ending visits at 37 weeks' gestation. The nurse then will perform a physical examination and assessment.

　　　　(a) Cardiovascular: Assess blood pressure, pulse rate (any irregularity of heart rate or palpitation, tachycardia). Assess for congestive heart failure, heart murmur.

　　　　(b) Respiratory: Auscultate client's lung sounds bilaterally for pulmonary edema, any abnormal breath sounds, rales, rhonchi, wheezes, and rate and rhythm.

　　　　(c) Musculoskeletal: Assess for edema, circulatory function (check pulses in all extremities), range of motion, any physical limitation.

　　　　(d) Gastrointestinal: Assess for abdominal distention, bowel sounds, and bowel movements. Instruct client on proper nutrition during pregnancy.

　　　　(e) Genitourinary: Assess for proper kidney function; watch for signs and symptoms of urinary tract infection, pyelonephritis, cystitis, etc. Increase fluid hydration and instruct client to keep a record of urinary output.

　　　　(f) Neurologic: Assess client for neurologic deficit, orientation to time, place, and person.

　　　　(g) Reproduction: Assess fetal movement, fetal heart tone, signs of labor (increase in contractions, bleeding, cramping, or rupture of membranes). Instruct client to notify physician immediately if any signs of labor occur.

　　　　(h) Metabolic: Watch for any signs of infection; record daily temperature.

　　　　(i) Head, ears, eyes, nose, throat (HEENT): Assess client for signs of periorbital edema, headaches, blurred vision, or any visual changes.

　　　　(j) Evaluate client's compliance with OB care provider orders.

      (k) If used, evaluate client's uterine monitoring system (how many contractions client has in 1 hour) and document.

   7) If used, home monitoring system is discontinued at 36 weeks' gestation.

   8) Home health aide requirements

      (a) Client is on bed rest with bathroom privileges.

      (b) Client receives no support from family or friends

      (c) Client lives alone

      (d) Client cannot stand for long periods

      (e) Client has other children that require care.

   9) The OB care provider is to provide any laboratory values and antenatal testing results to the perinatal nurse.

  10) Proper documentation of all conversations with OB care provider will be done by perinatal nurse.

Nursing Assessment

1. Activity
   a. Complete bed rest
   b. Bed rest with bathroom privileges
   c. Left lateral side exercises
   d. Passive range-of-motion exercises if ordered by OB care provider.
   e. Provide educational material concerning how to maintain bed rest during pregnancy;, for example, *Pregnancy at Bed Rest* by Susan H. Johnston and Deborah A. Kraut, St. Martin's Press, New York, 1990).
   f. Assess for any signs or symptoms of decreased circulation.
   g. Educate family regarding back rubs and frequent position changes.

2. Diet
   a. As per orders: Well-balanced diet with increased hydration

3. Education
   a. Educate client and family about premature labor.
   b. Provide emotional support to client and family.
   c. Provide information about support groups or other women with same diagnosis who can be called for reassurance.
   d. At 30 weeks' gestation, perinatal nurse will start instructing the client on childbirth education.

4. Medication

a. Educate client on the actions and side effects of each medication.

b. Review proper administration of medication during each nursing visit.

c. Review any new medication that client might be receiving for any contraindications of medications.

5. Follow-up Care

    a. Establish with client that after delivery, a follow-up appointment with her OB care provider is necessary.

    b. Encourage client to establish a yearly appointment with her OB care provider.

6. Individual Treatment Plan

    a. Level I: Preventive

        1) Nursing visits: Weekly visits can be decreased to once every other week.

        2) Home health aide: 3 to 5 days per week.

    b. Level II: Intermediate

        1) Nursing visits: 2 to 3 times per week for the first 2 to 3 weeks, then decreasing to once per week.

        2) Home health aide: 3 to 5 days a week.

    c. Level III: Acute

        1) Nursing visits: Daily visits starting day of referral. Weekly reports to OB care provider, or more frequently if there is a problem.

        2) Home health aide: 5 to 7 days per week. Maintain bed rest; prepare for premature labor, delivery, or possibly premature baby; introduce childbirth education.

■ PERINATAL HOME CARE PROTOCOL FOR PRETERM LABOR TREATED WITH TOCOLYTIC AGENTS

Eligibility

1. Identified as having had an episode of preterm labor

2. Required hospital intervention because of preterm labor

3. Stabilization of premature labor with tocolytics taken orally (PO) or by infusion pump

4. Laboratory values within normal limits

5. No signs of chorioamnionitis

A client will be discharged to home care only after stabilization on tocolytic medication. Once a client is considered at risk for premature labor, arrangements must be made for emergency transportation. If there is economic hardship, utilities companies also must be notified of a need for water, phone, and heat.

General Nursing and Treatment Orders

1. Predischarge evaluation (before day of discharge)

    a. History and physical assessment consisting of appropriate identifying information

        1) Name, address, phone number at location of client after discharge

        2) Referring OB provider, address and phone number

        3) Insurance type and number

        4) Obstetric history while in the hospital

            (a) Reaction to medication, what type of medication client received, and documented reaction.

            (b) Length of stay in labor and delivery department

            (c) Any special studies that occurred during hospitalization (eg, chest radiograph, electrocardiogram [ECG], and so forth)

            (d) Cervical dilation, effacement, and station

            (e) Fetal presentation

            (f) Results of ultrasound (level I and level II)

            (g) Gestational age or estimated date of confinement (EDC)

            (h) Cervical cultures

            (i) Amniocentesis lecithin-sphingomyelin (L/S) ratio

2. Socioeconomic evaluation

   a. Determine need for home health aide services.

      1) Obtain laboratory data and results of antenatal testing.

      2) Determine medication that will be prescribed for client at home.

   b. Plan of care

      1) After receiving referral from clinical administrator, nurse will make initial evaluation visit. The prenatal evaluation visit will include:

         (a) Physical and psychological assessment using the Prenatal Universal Home Risk Assessment tool. When combined with the information obtained from the Prenatal Data Collection and Risk Scoring Tool, this will help to determine appropriate level of care for home visiting patterns and interventions.

         (b) Complete obstetric, medical, and surgical history

         (c) Social and economic assessment

         (d) Establish whether the client needs a home health aide or any other community resources.

      2) The perinatal nurse will set up a plan of care with referring OB care provider, the client, and the insurer if indicated.

      3) The perinatal nurse will communicate plan of treatment to the clinical administrator.

      4) The perinatal nurse will establish the specific day for nursing visits with the client.

2. Nursing assessment with each visit

   a. The perinatal nurse will perform a complete physical assessment to include:

      1) Cardiovascular: Assess blood pressure; watch for hypotension; pulse rate (tachycardia, irregular heart rate); abnormal heart sounds suggesting congestive heart failure. Check for substernal chest pain.

      2) Respiratory: Auscultate lungs for rate, rhythm, abnormal breath (rales, rhonchi, wheezes) to note any signs of pulmonary edema.

      3) Metabolic: Assess client's temperature, test urine for glucose (watch for hypoglycemia and hyperglycemia), monitor client's hemoglobin and hematocrit, monitor serum potassium levels (hypokalemia).

      4) Gastrointestinal: Assess for signs of nausea, vomiting, diarrhea, or any gastrointestinal disturbances.

      5) Genitourinary: Watch for signs of fluid retention, decrease in urination, concentration of urine.

      6) Musculoskeletal: Watch for signs of fluid retention, check for edema of extremities (pitting or nonpitting); assess for signs of decreased circulation.

      7) Neurologic: Watch for signs of nervousness, tremors, dizziness, headaches, and blurred vision.

        8) Psychological: Assess client's emotional status; encourage client to express concerns and problems related to pregnancy complications, outcome, and activity restrictions.

        9) Reproductive: Assess any contractions (frequency, duration, and intensity). If contractions have increased, notify OB care provider. Perform cervical examination as per OB care provider orders (for assessment of further dilation, engagement, effacement).

        10) Fetal: Assess fetal heart rate (should be between 120 and 160 beats/min) and fetal movement.

    b. The perinatal nurse also will assess:

        1) Client's understanding of prescribed tocolytic therapy (dosage, frequency, side effects) and compliance with therapy

        2) Client's understanding of activity restrictions and compliance with restrictions

        3) Client's knowledge of signs and symptoms of preterm labor

        4) Client's understanding of strategies to reduce the risk of preterm labor

    c. The perinatal nurse will perform other activities as ordered in the plan of care.

3. Communication with OB care provider

    a. The perinatal nurse will communicate weekly or as needed with the OB care provider on the progress of the client.

    b. Any clinical laboratory values, changes in cervical examination, or results from antenatal testing will be available for the perinatal nurse.

    c. Every 30 days, the OB care provider will be required to review and update the plan of treatment.

Nursing Assessment

1. Activity

    a. Complete bed rest or bed rest with bathroom privileges (left lateral position).

    b. Passive range-of-motion exercises if ordered by OB care provider.

2. Diet

    a. Balanced diet

        1) Increased fiber

        2) Increased fluid: 6 to 8 glasses a day

        3) Increased protein

3. Education

    a. Education of client and family members about preterm labor

        1) What is a contraction? Self-palpation, timing of contractions

        2) Signs and symptoms of preterm labor

3) Notifying OB care provider if increase in contractions or other signs and symptoms of preterm labor

b. Educate client concerning action, dosage, frequency, and side effects of tocolytic agents.

c. Teach client uterine self-palpation.

d. Teach client to count fetal movements.

e. Offer practical information for dealing with pregnancy bed rest (eg, *Pregnancy at Bed Rest,* by Susan H. Johnston and Deborah A. Kraut, St. Martin's Press, New York, 1990).

f. Prepare client for preterm delivery and caring for premature infant.

1) Educational material on premature delivery and premature infants (eg, Helen Harrison's *Premature Baby Book,* St. Martin's Press, New York, 1983).

g. Provide emotional support.

1) Perinatal nurse listens to client concerns, providing information about client's diagnosis and positive reinforcement.

2) Support groups: Establish a phone connection with other clients at home in premature labor as well as with other clients who have experienced premature labor with a positive outcome.

h. Provide client with childbirth education classes at 30 weeks' gestation.

i. Offer information about passive range-of-motion exercises if ordered by OB care provider.

j. Educate client and family regarding position changes and comfort measures for bed rest (back rubs).

4. Medication

a. Educate client regarding the action, dosage, frequency, and side effects of each medication.

b. Review any new medication that client might be receiving for any contraindications.

5. Follow-up care

a. Establish with client that after delivery, a follow-up appointment with her health care provider is necessary for both mother and baby.

b. Encourage client to establish a yearly appointment with her OB/GYN care provider.

6. Individual treatment plan

a. Level I: Preventive

1) Nursing visits: Weekly visits can be decreased to every other week.

2) Home health aide: 3 to 5 times per week

b. Level II: Intermediate

1) Nursing visits: 2 to 3 times weekly for first 2 to 3 weeks, then decreasing to once per week.

2) Home health aide: 3 to 5 days per week.

c. Level III: Acute

    1) Nursing visits: Daily visits starting day of referral. Weekly reports to OB care provider, or more frequently if there is a problem. Maintain bed rest; prepare for premature labor, delivery, or possibly premature baby; introduce childbirth education.

    2) Home health aide: 5 to 7 times per week.

■ PERINATAL HOME CARE PROTOCOL FOR PREECLAMPSIA (MILD)

Eligibility

1. History of preeclampsia with prior pregnancy.

2. No renal disease or oliguria (400 mL in 24 hours).

3. Slight increase in proteinuria, but not to exceed 5 g in 24 hours or +3 or +4 with dip stick)

4. No neurologic changes

5. If in hospital: stabilization of blood pressure, nonelevated laboratory values

6. Referral form from OB care provider, with information regarding first examination results for hypertension, proteinuria, weight gain, increased edema

Once a client is identified as high risk by using the Prenatal Data Collection and Risk Scoring Tool, arrangements must be made for emergency transportation.

General Nursing and Treatment Orders

1. Plan of care
   a. Information to be received at time of referral, if available:
      1) Socioeconomic evaluation
      2) Laboratory tests
      3) Antenatal test results
      4) Complete physical assessment and history
         (a) Medical and surgical history
         (b) Past and current obstetric history
         (c) Identifying information such as client's name, address, and phone number; referring OB care provider, address and phone number; insurance type and number; known drug allergies; any medications prescribed; type of home care, visits, and frequency expected.
   b. Establishing plan of care with short- and long-term goals.
      1) Classification of preeclamptic and eclamptic client
         (a) Mild: Mean arterial pressure (MAP) is less than 106 mmHg (140/90) with an increase in diastolic pressure of more than 20 mmHg on two occasions 6 hours apart with the client at bed rest; proteinuria, edema, or both develop; this defini-

tion requires accurate knowledge of the client's blood pressure (BP) readings before pregnancy.

(b) Moderate: MAP is greater than 107 mmHg (140/90) and less than 126 mmHg (160/110), or an increase in BP of greater than 30 mmHg systolic or 20 mmHg diastolic; this increase in BP is combined with appreciable proteinuria, and edema of the lower extremities is usually, but not always, present.

(c) Severe: MAP exceeds 126 mmHg (160/110) at least two occasions 6 hours apart with the client at bed rest, and urinary protein is greater than 5 g per 24 hours; usually accompanied by headaches and blurred vision; if right upper quadrant or epigastric pain, oliguria, pulmonary edema, or visual or cerebral disturbances occur, severe disease is present; edema of the face, hands, and lower extremities is usually present.

(d) Eclampsia: This consists of generalized seizures accompanied by hypertension and proteinuria in a pregnant client; other causes of seizure must be excluded; the seizures may occur postpartally as well as antepartally.

2. Perinatal nursing visit

a. The clinical administrator assigns a perinatal nurse to complete an initial prenatal evaluation visit.

1) A nursing visit is made as prescribed by OB care provider within 72 hours after referral, and findings are reported to provider.

2) The prenatal evaluation visit will include

(a) Physical and psychological assessment using the Prenatal Universal Home Risk Assessment Tool, which, combined with the information obtained from the Prenatal Data Collection and Risk Scoring Tool, will help to determine the appropriate level of care for home visiting patterns and interventions.

b. If severe preeclampsia is present, daily visits are made until the client is stabilized.

c. Home health aide services are evaluated by nurse at first visit in the home.

d. Physical assessments are made as follows:

1) Cardiovascular: Assess blood pressure, both lying down and sitting up, in left arm; if elevated, lay client in left lateral position; assess apical heart rate for regularity, rhythm, and sound; assess client for congestive heart failure.

2) Respiratory: Assess client's lungs for pulmonary edema, any abnormal breath sounds, rate, and rhythm.

3) Musculoskeletal: Assess for edema, circulatory function (check pedal pulses), range of motion; maintain bed rest with bathroom privileges and lying on left side.

4) Gastrointestinal: Assess for abdominal distention, bowel sounds, and bowel movement; instruct client on nutrition for increased protein in diet.

    5) Genitourinary: Assess kidney function and watch for signs of oliguria (output of 500 mL or less in a 24-hour period); instruct client on keeping a record of intake and output; assess for proteinuria.

    6) Neurologic: Assess for orientation, hyperreflexia, petechiae.

    7) Reproductive: Assess fetal movements, fetal heart tones, and signs of labor, rupture of membranes, cramping and bleeding; instruct client on taking fetal movement counts and self-palpation to detect uterine contractions.

    8) Metabolic: Watch for signs of infection; record temperature.

    9) HEENT: Assess for signs of periorbital edema, dizziness, spots before eyes, headaches, and blurred vision.

  e. Antenatal testing to be tracked through plan of care

    1) Ultrasound (level I or level II)

    2) Doppler flow studies

    3) Biophysical profiles

    4) Non-stress test

    5) Oxytocin challenge test

    6) 24-hour urine collection

  f. OB care provider

    1) Communication and documentation of all conversations with OB care provider must be done by perinatal nurse.

    2) At a maximum interval of every 30 days, the plan of treatment must be reviewed and updated by OB care provider.

Nursing Assessment

1. Activity

  a. Bed rest with bathroom privileges; client advised to lie on left side

2. Diet

  a. High-protein diet

  b. Recommended dietary allowance of sodium

3. Education

  a. Instruct client on fetal movement counts and uterine self-palpation.

  b. Educate client on signs and symptoms of increasing hypertension—preeclampsia:

    1) Increased edema

    2) Increased protein in urine

    3) Headaches, dizziness, blurred vision

      4) Increased weight gain

      5) Decrease in urine output

      6) Increase in blood pressure

      7) Check for hyperreflexia

  c. Instruct family member(s) on how to take client's blood pressure.

  d. Teach client to record an accurate intake and output of fluids.

  e. Prepare client for delivery of child. Teach client childbirth education classes at home if condition prohibits attendance at classes given in the community.

  f. Teach client deep breathing and relaxation techniques.

  g. Reinforce with client the actions and side effects of any medication taken.

  h. Teach client about recording weights daily (same time each day)

  i. Teach client about seizure precautions: padded tongue blade by bedside

4. Medication

  a. Educate client on the actions and side effects of each medication.

  b. Review at each nursing visit proper administration of medication.

  c. Review any new medication that client might be receiving for contraindications.

5. Follow-up care

  a. Establish with client that after delivery, follow-up appointment with health care provider is necessary for her and baby.

  b. Encourage client to establish a yearly appointment for her OB/GYN care provider.

6. Individual treatment plan

  a. Level I: Preventive

      1) Nursing visits: Weekly visits; can be decreased to once every other week

      2) Home health aide: 3 to 5 days per week

  b. Level II: Intermediate

      1) Nursing visits: 2 to 3 times a week for first 2 to 3 weeks, then decreasing to once per week

      2) Home health aide: 3 to 5 days per week

  c. Level III: Acute

      1) Nursing visits: Daily visits starting day of referral. Weekly reports to OB care provider, or if problem, more frequently. Maintain bed rest; prepare for premature labor, delivery, or possibly premature baby; introduce childbirth education.

      2) Home health aide: 5 to 7 days per week

PERINATAL HOME CARE PROTOCOL FOR PREGNANCY-INDUCED HYPERTENSION

Eligibility

1. Increase in blood pressure to above 140/90 mmHg after 20 weeks of pregnancy

2. Obesity or poor nutrition

3. Family history of hypertension or vascular disease

4. Diabetic mothers

5. Women who have experienced pregnancy-induced hypertension (PIH) in previous pregnancies

6. Women with multiple fetuses, hydramnios, large fetus, or fetal hydrops

Once a client has been identified as a high risk by using the Prenatal Data Collection and Risk Scoring Tool, arrangements must be made for emergency transportation.

General Nursing and Treatment Orders

1. Initial perinatal nursing visit referred by OB care provider
   a. Before nursing visit, the following information is received from OB care provider:
      1) Client's name, address, and phone number
      2) Referring physician, address, and phone number
      3) Insurance type and number
      4) Known drug allergies
      5) Any medication client is taking
      6) Type of home care; frequency of visits
      7) Socioeconomic status of client
      8) Antenatal test results
      9) Past medical/obstetric history
      10) Present obstetric course

2. Perinatal nurse visit
   a. The clinical administrator will assign a perinatal nurse to make an initial home evaluation. The prenatal evaluation will include:
      1) Physical and psychosocial assessment using Prenatal Universal Home Risk Assessment tool
      2) Determination of need for home health service, providing physical assessment
         (a) Cardiovascular: Assess blood pressure in left arm both lying down and sitting up;

      if elevated, lay client on left side; assess apical heart rate for regularity, rhythm, and sound; assess client for congestive heart failure.

  (b) Respiratory: Assess client's lungs for pulmonary edema, any abnormal breath sounds, rate, and rhythm.

  (c) Musculoskeletal: Assess for edema, circulatory function (check pedal pulses), range of motion; maintain bed rest with bathroom privileges and lying on left side.

  (d) Gastrointestinal: Assess for abdominal distention, bowel sounds, and bowel movement; instruct client on nutrition for increased protein in diet.

  (e) Genitourinary: Assess kidney function and watch for signs of oliguria (output of 500 mL or less in a 24-hour period); instruct client on keeping a record of intake and output; assess for proteinuria.

  (f) Neurologic: Assess for orientation, hyperreflexia, petechiae.

  (g) Reproductive: Assess fetal movements, teach uterine self-palpation, fetal heart tones, signs of labor, rupture of membranes, cramping and bleeding; instruct client on taking fetal movement counts.

  (h) Metabolic: Watch for signs of infection; record temperature.

  (i) HEENT: Assess for signs of periorbital edema, dizziness, spots before eyes, headaches, and blurred vision.

3. Antenatal testing that should be tracked through plan of care

  a. Before 28 weeks: Ultrasound to rule out intrauterine growth retardation (IUGR)/oligohydramnios

  b. After 28 weeks

    1) Ultrasounds—watch biparietal diameters

    2) Fetal movements: Normal fetal movements peak in afternoon and evening; fetal movements should be assessed by the client within the first hour after meals for 1 hour; there should be 8 to 10 movements

    3) Non-stress test (NST)

    4) Oxytocin challenge test (OCT) or nipple stimulation challenge test (NSCT)

    5) Amniocentesis—should be started at 30 to 36 weeks, depending on maternal disease

    6) Biophysical profiles

    7) Doppler flow studies

4. OB Care Provider

  a. Communication and documentation of all conversations with OB care provider must be done by perinatal nurse.

  b. At a minimum of every 30 days, the plan of treatment must be reviewed and updated.

Nursing Assessment

1. Activity

    a. Bed rest with bathroom privileges; lie on left side

2. Diet

    a. High-protein diet.

    b. Recommended dietary allowance of sodium

    c. Fluid intake of 6 to 8 glasses per day

3. Education

    a. Instruct client regarding fetal movements and using uterine self-palpation to detect premature labor contractions.

    b. Educate client on signs and symptoms of increasing hypertension—preeclampsia:

        1) Increased edema

        2) Increased protein in urine

        3) Headaches, dizziness, blurred vision

        4) Increased weight gain

        5) Decrease in urine output

        6) Increase in blood pressure

    c. Instruct family member on taking client's blood pressure.

    d. Teach client to record an accurate intake and output of fluids.

    e. Prepare client for delivery of child, if client cannot attend childbirth education classes.

    f. Teach client deep-breathing and relaxation techniques.

    g. Reinforce with client actions and side effects of any medication that is being ingested.

    h. Teach client to record daily weights (same time each day)

4. Medication

    a. Educate client on the actions and side effects of each medication.

    b. Review with each nursing visit proper administration of medication.

    c. Review any new medication that client might be receiving for any contraindications of medications.

5. Follow-up care

    a. Establish with client that after delivery, a follow-up appointment with health care provider is necessary for her and her baby.

    b. Encourage client to establish a yearly appointment with her OB/GYN provider.

6. Nursing visit plan

    a. Level I: Preventive

        1) Nursing visits: Weekly visits; can be decreased to once every other week

        2) Home health aide: 3 to 5 days per week

    b. Level II: Intermediate

        1) Nursing visits: 2 to 3 times per week for first 2 to 3 weeks, then decreasing to once per week

        2) Home health aide: 3 to 5 days per week

    c. Level III: Acute

        1) Nursing visits: Daily visits starting day of referral. Weekly reports to physician, or if there is a problem, more frequently. Maintain bed rest; prepare for premature labor, delivery, or possibly premature baby; introduce childbirth education

        2) Home health aide: 5 to 7 days per week

▓ PERINATAL HOME CARE PROTOCOL FOR CHRONIC HYPERTENSION IN PREGNANCY

Eligibility

1. Blood pressure above 140/90 mmHg detected in a client earlier than 20 weeks or prepregnancy

2. Medical history of hypertension
   a. No proteinuria
   b. Not characterized within the high risk group
   c. No renal disease
   d. No signs of preeclampsia early in pregnancy
   e. Notification of appropriate utilities companies for water, phone, and heat if there is economic hardship.

Once a client is identified as high risk using the Prenatal Data Collection and Risk Scoring Tool, arrangements must be made for emergency transportation. These clients will be initiated into the program at the first prenatal visit.

General Nursing and Treatment Orders

1. Initial prenatal visit by OB care provider
   a. Client is identified as either high risk or low risk
      1) Characteristics of clients in high risk group include:
         (a) Maternal age: 30 years
         (b) Duration of hypertension: 15 years
         (c) Blood pressure greater than 160/110 mmHg early in pregnancy
         (d) Diabetes (classes B through F)
         (e) Cardiomyopathy
         (f) Renal disease
         (g) Connective tissue disease
         (h) Previous thromboembolism
         (i) Previous severe preeclampsia early in pregnancy
         (j) Previous abruptio placentae
      2) Characteristics of clients in low risk group include:
         (a) Blood pressure equal to 140/90 mmHg on two occasions 24 hours apart
         (b) Previously on antihypertensive medication
         (c) Previously on diuretics
         (d) No renal disease

    (e) No diabetes

    (f) Maternal age older than 30 years

    (g) Duration of hypertension longer than 15 years

    (h) No history of severe preeclampsia or eclampsia

b. Once the client has been identified as a low risk client, the OB care provider will initiate a referral to the antepartum program.

c. Before initial perinatal nursing visit, the obstetrician will provide the following information:

    1) Chest x-ray results

    2) Electrocardiogram results

    3) Laboratory data

    4) Ultrasound results

    5) Biophysical profile results

    6) Medical history

    7) Previous and current obstetric history

2. Perinatal nursing visit

a. Socioeconomic evaluation

    1) Documenting information from obstetrician on perinatal chart

b. Complete physical assessment using Prenatal Universal Home Risk Assessment tool

    1) Cardiovascular: Assess blood pressure, both lying down and sitting up, in left arm; if elevated, place client on left side; assess apical heart rate for regularity, rhythm, and sound; assess client for congestive heart failure.

    2) Respiratory: Assess client's lungs for pulmonary edema, any abnormal breath sounds, rate, and rhythm.

    3) Musculoskeletal: Assess for edema, circulatory function (check pedal pulses), range of motion; maintain bed rest with bathroom privileges and lying on left side.

    4) Gastrointestinal: Assess for abdominal distention, bowel sounds, and bowel movement; instruct client about nutrition for increased protein in diet.

    5) Genitourinary: Assess kidney function and watch for signs of oliguria (output of 500 mL or less in a 24-hour period); instruct client on keeping a record on intake and output; assess for proteinuria.

    6) Neurologic: Assess for orientation, hyperreflexia, petechiae.

    7) Reproductive: Assess fetal movements, teach uterine self-palpation, fetal heart tones, signs of labor, rupture of membranes, cramping and bleeding; instruct client on taking fetal movement counts.

    8) Metabolic: Watch for signs of infection; record temperature.

    9) HEENT: Assess for signs of periorbital edema, dizziness, spots before eyes, headaches, and blurred vision.

  c. Complete maternal history

    1) Allergies, current medication

    2) Medical and obstetric history

  d. Nurse on call 24 hours a day

  e. Frequency of nursing visits: 3 times per week

  f. Home health aide evaluation (Does client have the necessary support system to maintain bed rest?)

3. Antenatal testing information that should be tracked through plan of care.

  a. Before 28 weeks: Ultrasound to evaluate for intrauterine growth retardation (IUGR)/oligohydramnios

  b. After 28 weeks:

    1) Ultrasound: Watch biparietal diameters

    2) Fetal movements: Normal fetal movements peak in afternoon and evening; fetal movements should be assessed by the client within the first hour after meals for 1 hour; there should be 8 to 10 movements.

    3) Non-stress test (NST)

    4) Oxytocin challenge test (OCT) or nipple stimulation challenge test (NSCST)

    5) Amniocentesis: Should be performed at 30 to 36 weeks, depending on maternal disease

    6) Biophysical profiles

    7) Doppler flow studies

4. OB care provider

  a. Communication and documentation of all conversations with OB care provider must be done by perinatal nurse.

  b. At a minimum of every 30 days, the plan of treatment must be reviewed and updated.

Nursing Assessment

1. Activity

  a. No limitations at beginning of pregnancy for low risk group

  b. High risk group: Bed rest with bathroom privileges or reduced activity

  c. Lying on left side to increase placental perfusion

  d. If low risk client becomes more hypertensive, then activities of daily living (ADL) would be limited.

2. Diet
   a. Increase protein
   b. Decrease sodium intake
   c. General diet

3. Education
   a. Instruct client on fetal movement counts and uterine self-palpation to detect premature labor contractions.
   b. Educate client on signs and symptoms of increasing hypertension—preeclampsia:
      1) Increased edema
      2) Increased protein in urine
      3) Headaches, dizziness, blurred vision
      4) Increase in weight gain
      5) Decrease in urine output if increase in blood pressure
   c. Instruct family members how to take client's blood pressure.
   d. Teach client to take an accurate record of fluid intake and output.
   e. Prepare client for delivery of child, if client cannot attend childbirth education classes.
   f. Teach client deep breathing and relaxation techniques.
   g. Reinforce with client actions and side effects of any medication that is being ingested.
   h. Teach client to record daily weights (same time each day)

4. Medication
   a. Educate client on the actions and side effects of each medication.
   b. Review at each nursing visit the proper administration of medication.
   c. Review any new medication that client might be receiving for any contraindications of medications.

5. Follow-up care
   a. Establish with client that after delivery, a follow-up appointment with her health care provider is necessary for her and her baby.
   b. Encourage client to establish a yearly appointment with her OB care provider.

6. Individual Treatment Plan
   a. Level I: Preventive
      1) Nursing visits: Weekly visits; can be decreased to once every other week.
      2) Home health aide: 3 to 5 days per week
   b. Level II: Intermediate
      1) Nursing visits: 2 to 3 times per week for first 2 to 3 weeks, then decreasing to once per week.
      2) Home health aide: 3 to 5 days per week.

c. Level III: Acute

    1) Nursing visits: Daily visits starting day of referral. Weekly reports to physician, or if there is a problem, more frequently. Maintain bed rest; prepare for premature labor, delivery, or possibly premature baby; introduce childbirth education.

    2) Home health aide: 5 to 7 days per week.

▮ PERINATAL HOME CARE PROTOCOL FOR GESTATIONAL DIABETES IN PREGNANCY

Eligibility

1. Clients with impaired glucose tolerance test

2. Family history of diabetes

3. Pregnancies with unexplained stillbirth or delivery of macrosomic infants

4. No vascular disease

5. Condition is diet-controlled

6. Risks identified through use of Prenatal Data Collection and Risk Scoring Tool.

General Nursing and Treatment Orders

1. Before perinatal nursing visit:
   a. OB care provider's identification of gestational diabetes, using White's Classification of Diabetes in Pregnancy (see Appendix)
      1) Class A: Diabetes appearing during pregnancy but absent in the nonpregnant state (most often restricted to clients with abnormal GTT and excluding those with elevated fasting blood sugar [FBS]).
      2) Class B: Overt diabetes, onset after age 20 years, duration of less than 10 years; no vascular disease
      3) Class C: Onset between age of 10 and 20 years or duration of 10 to 19 years; no vascular disease
      4) Class D: Onset before age of 10 years or duration of more than 10 years; benign retinopathy
      5) Class E: Calcification present in pelvic vessels (this category is no longer used by most authorities)
      6) Class F: Diabetic nephropathy, proteinuria, decreased creatinine clearance
      7) Class R: Proliferative retinopathy
      8) Class RF: Nephropathy plus retinopathy
      9) Class H: Arteriosclerotic heart disease

    b. Detections of gestational diabetes via GTT

        1) Scale of glucose tolerance test

            (a) 1 hour = 190

            (b) 2 hours = 165

            (c) 3 hours = 145

    c. Obtain diagnostic data from OB care provider.

        1) Ultrasound for gestational age

        2) Presence of glycosuria, ketonuria, or proteinuria

    d. Obtain baseline vital signs

    e. Review of antepartum history for predisposing factors

    f. Obtain appropriate identifying information

        1) Client's name, address, phone number

        2) Referring provider's name, address, phone number

        3) Insurance type and number

        4) Known drug allergies

        5) Type of home care, visits, and frequency anticipated

            (a) Client to be seen at least biweekly until 36 weeks, but level of care is more appropriately determined after use of Prenatal Universal Home Risk Assessment tool at the initial home visit

    g. Socioeconomic evaluation

2. Perinatal nursing visit

    a. The clinical administrator will assign a perinatal nurse to make an initial home evaluation. The prenatal evaluation will include:

        1) Physical and psychosocial assessment using Prenatal Universal Home Risk Assessment tool

        2) Determination of need for home health services

    b. System assessment:

        1) Cardiovascular: Assess blood pressure, apical pulse (rhythm and sound)

        2) Respiratory: Assess lung fields, respiratory rate

        3) Musculoskeletal: Assess for range of motion of extremities

        4) Gastrointestinal: Proper nutritional intake, watch for signs/symptoms of nausea or vomiting

        5) Genitourinary: Watch for polyuria; assess glucose in urine

        6) Neurologic: Blurred vision, headaches, dizziness (orthostatic)

        7) Reproductive: Assess fetal heart tones, assess and teach uterine palpation, fetal movement, fundal height

8) Metabolic: Blood sugar elevation (teach how to use dextro-stix); temperature (increase in temperature, questionable infection that would increase glucose)

9) Skin: Assess for warm and dry skin

Nursing Assessment

1. Activity: No limitations out of bed

2. Diet

    a. Provide dietary counseling.

    b. Diet should contain 30 to 35 calories/kg actual body weight.

3. Education

    a. Proper nutritional counseling

    b. Educate client and family members concerning diabetes in pregnancy.

       1) Explain signs and symptoms of hypoglycemia and hyperglycemia.

       2) Teach client how to monitor glucose in urine.

       3) Teach client how to monitor serum glucose.

    c. Prepare client for childbirth education.

    d. Teach client how to keep daily record of fetal movement count and uterine self-palpation to detect premature labor contractions.

4. Medication

    a. Educate client about the actions and side effects of each medication.

    b. Review at each nursing visit proper administration of medication.

    c. Review any new medication that client might be receiving for any contraindications.

5. Follow-up care

    a. Establish with client that after delivery, a follow-up appointment with her health care provider is necessary for her and her baby.

    b. Encourage client to establish a yearly appointment with her OB care provider.

6. Individual Treatment Plan

    a. Level I: Preventive

       1) Nursing visits: Weekly visits; can be decreased to once every other week

       2) Home health aide: 3 to 5 days per week

    b. Level II: Intermediate

       1) Nursing visits: 2 to 3 times per week for first 2 to 3 weeks, then decreasing to once per week

       2) Home health aide: 3 to 5 days per week

   c. Level III: Acute

      1) Nursing visits: Daily visits starting day of referral. Weekly reports to physician, or if there is a problem, more frequently. Maintain bed rest; prepare for premature labor, delivery, or possibly premature baby; introduce childbirth education.

      2) Home health aide: 5 to 7 days per week

■ PERINATAL HOME CARE PROTOCOL FOR DIABETES IN PREGNANCY

The goal of antepartum management is maintaining euglycemia between 60 and 120 mg/dL throughout each 24-hour period on an outpatient basis.

Eligibility

1. Insulin-dependent diabetes mellitus or gestational diabetes

2. Versed in administration of insulin, if insulin dependent

3. Monitoring glucose level with a glucose oxidase–impregnated reagent strip as well as glucose reflectance meter

4. Reactive NST

5. Consultation with endocrinologist or perinatologist

6. Normal fetal growth with serial ultrasound

7. No abnormal laboratory values

8. Dietary consultation

9. Identification of high risk using Prenatal Data Collection and Risk Scoring Tool

General Nursing and Treatment Orders

1. Before perinatal nursing visit
   a. Obtain obstetric, medical, surgical, and psychosocial assessment from OB care provider.
   b. Determine diabetes classification and type and current management, which includes dietary needs, glucose monitoring, and daily insulin requirements.
      1) White's Classification of Diabetes Mellitus (DM) and other categories of glucose tolerance:
         (a) Class A: Diabetes appearing during pregnancy but absent in the nonpregnant state (most often restricted to clients with abnormal GTT and excluding those with elevated FBS)
         (b) Class B: Overt diabetes, onset after age 20 years, duration less than 10 years; no vascular disease
         (c) Class C: Onset between age of 10 and 20 years or duration of 10 to 19 years; no vascular disease
         (d) Class D: Onset before age of 10 years or duration more than 10 years; benign retinopathy

(e) Class E: Calcification present in pelvic vessels (this category no longer used by most authorities)

(f) Class F: Diabetic nephropathy, proteinuria, decreased creatinine clearance

(g) Class R: Proliferative retinopathy

(h) Class RF: Nephropathy plus retinopathy

(i) Class H: Arteriosclerotic heart disease

2) Types of diabetes mellitus

(a) Type I, insulin-dependent (IDDM).

(b) Type II, non–insulin-dependent (NIDDM): Non-obese NIDDM and obese NIDDM.

(c) Secondary diabetes

(d) Impaired glucose tolerance (IGT)

(e) Type III, gestational diabetes (GDM)

(f) Type IV, secondary diabetes (conditions/symptoms associated with IGT)

2. Perinatal nursing visit

a. The clinical administrator will assign a perinatal nurse to complete an initial evaluation visit. Prenatal home visit will include:

1) Physical and psychosocial assessment using Prenatal Universal Home Risk Assessment tool

b. Nursing visits should be anticipated to be a minimum of 3 to 5 times per week for the first few weeks, then decrease as per OB care provider's orders, but the most appropriate level of care is determined through the use of the Prenatal Universal Home Risk Assessment tool after the initial home visit. See Nursing Care Plan: Diabetes Mellitus on page XXX.

c. Establish maintenance control of maternal blood sugar between 60 and 120 mg/dL.

d. Identify other controlling factors of diabetes, such as:

1) Severity of the disease state (see White's classifications)

2) Emotional condition

3) Activity level

4) Dietary factors: Compliance or resistance

5) Insulin dosage

6) Infection: Commonly results in insulin resistance and ketoacidosis if not recognized and treated

7) Nausea and vomiting may lead to insulin shock or to insulin resistance if starvation is severe enough to cause ketosis.

8) Socioeconomic hardship

e. A total nursing physical assessment is to be done with each nursing visit.

1) Cardiovascular: Assess blood pressure, pulse, watch for signs of hypertension.

2) Respiratory: Assess breath sounds in all lung fields for any congestion or abnormal breath sounds; assess rate and lung expansion.

3) Metabolic: Assess client record of glucose in blood, glucose and ketones in urine; insulin administration.

4) Gastrointestinal: Assess calorie American Diabetes Association diet, assess for nausea and vomiting.

5) Genitourinary: Assess for signs and symptoms of urinary tract infection (UTI).

6) Reproductive: Assess for signs of labor, rupture of membranes, cramping and bleeding; obtain from obstetrician serial ultrasound and NST results; watch for increased uterine growth suggesting macrosomia. Assess and teach client how to maintain appropriate track of fetal movements and uterine palpation to assess for signs of premature labor contractions.

7) Neurologic: Assess for signs of blurred vision, double vision, lethargy, change in level of consciousness.

8) Musculoskeletal: Assess circulatory function (check pulses) and range of motion.

9) Fetal: Assess fetal heart rate and fetal movement.

10) Psychological: Assess client's emotional status, encourage client to express concerns and problems related to pregnancy complications, and outcome.

  f. Insulin requirements should be adjusted by a consulting endocrinologist or perinatologist.

  g. Antepartum fetal testing should be tracked through course of care.

1) Ultrasound testing

2) Fetal movements: Daily surveillance beginning at 24 weeks' gestation

3) Biophysical profile for class A—Type II, B, C, and D diabetics. This is started near 32 weeks and done weekly until delivery. If disease is complicated or advanced, it is started by weeks 26 to 28. For Class A—Type I, it is done at 38 to 40 weeks.

4) Contraction stress test: Usually done if biophysical profile is not available (done as inpatient).

5) NST: Usually done weekly

6) Doppler umbilical cord artery study: Used to determine Intrauterine Growth Retardation

7) Amniocentesis: To determine L/S ratio for lung maturity, prevent respiratory distress syndrome (RDS). Usually done after 38 weeks.

3. Goals of client Care Management

  a. Non—insulin-dependent gestational diabetes

1) Nutritional counseling

2) Glucose monitoring

3) Compliance with medical follow-up

  b. Insulin-dependent diabetes mellitus (IDDM)

   1) Home monitoring and control consists of multiple facets:

    (a) Blood glucose monitoring is done 2 to 10 times per day as per physician's order.

    (b) Blood glucose sample (BGS) should be taken before meals and snacks, 2 hours after meals, and at bedtime (the first BGS is considered the fasting blood sugar [FBS]).

    (c) Teach the client how to perform dextrostix method for testing blood glucose level. Adhere to standard precautions.

   2) Urine testing for ketones

    (a) Test for ketones on first void of day, 2 to 4 times per week. If ketonuria is present in two consecutive specimens, report this to the OB care provider.

    (b) Glucose: sugar in the urine is not used as a reliable means of determining management because of lower renal threshold during pregnancy.

   3) Insulin management

    (a) Type of insulin: Usually biosynthetic human insulin

    (b) Insulin classification: Rapid and intermediate-acting insulin is used during pregnancy.

   4) Insulin dosage is calculated according to trimester on 24-hour basis.

    (a) The first increased insulin need usually occurs between 10 and 14 weeks of pregnancy; the second increase occurs between 28 and 32 weeks of pregnancy; then it gradually increases until delivery.

    (b) For gestational diabetics: the 24-hour insulin dosage may be given in one injection before breakfast, but for most pregnant IDDM women, multiple doses are necessary to achieve control.

    (c) The 24-hour dose is divided so 66% to 75% of total is given in the morning, and the remaining is given before the evening meal. If blood sugars are hyperglycemic, additional insulin may be necessary (regular insulin).

    (d) Insulin pump: Administered through infusion pump to avoid multiple subcutaneous injections. Only recommended if client cannot achieve goals. The bolus of insulin is delivered before meals.

Nursing Assessment

1. Activity

 a. Exercise improves insulin sensitivity. Should be done only on physician's recommendation and based on severity of DM.

2. Diet

a. Caloric needs are determined by the weight of the client. Generally a 25-pound weight gain and intake of 2,000 to 2,400 calories per day is recommended.

b. Nutritional Balance

    1) 50% to 60% calories from carbohydrates

    2) 12% to 20% calories from proteins

    3) 20% to 30% calories from fat

    4) High fiber

    5) Increased fluid intake

c. Meal and snack pattern can be individualized. Example: Three meals and evening snack = 25% calories at breakfast, 30% at lunch, 30% at dinner, 15% at bedtime; or five to seven smaller meals per day.

3. Education

a. Teach client and family signs and symptoms of hypoglycemia and hyperglycemia.

b. Teach client medication dosage, frequency, action, side effects, and contraindications.

c. Teach how to maintain daily record of fetal movement counts and uterine self-palpation.

4. Follow-up

a. Establish follow-up appointment schedule with perinatologist or endocrinologist.

5. Individual treatment plan

a. Level I: Preventive

    1) Nursing visits: Weekly visits; can be decreased to once every other week

    2) Home health aide: 3 to 5 days per week

b. Level II: Intermediate

    1) Nursing visits: 2 to 3 times per week for first 2 to 3 weeks, then decreasing to once per week

    2) Home health aide: 3 to 5 days per week

c. Level III: Acute

    1) Nursing visits: Daily visits starting day of referral. Weekly reports to OB care provider or, if there is a problem, more frequently. Maintain bed rest; prepare for premature labor, delivery, or possibly premature baby; introduce childbirth education.

    2) Home health aide: 5 to 7 days per week

▇ PERINATAL HOME CARE PROTOCOL FOR PLACENTA PREVIA (MARGINAL OR PARTIAL)

Eligibility

1. Diagnosis of marginal or partial previa by ultrasound

2. Stabilization of laboratory values: hemoglobin, hematocrit, fibrinogen, coagulation studies

3. Free of infection

4. On complete bed rest with or without bathroom privileges

5. Preliminary risk assessment completed through use of the Prenatal Data Collection and Risk Scoring Tool

6. Home monitoring system in place if ordered by OB care provider

7. Perinatal support team

Arrangements will need to be made for emergency transportation or accommodations in a hotel if necessary to be located within a safe distance from the hospital. Hospital accommodations may even be necessary if the obstetrician determines that the client lives too far from the institution. It also may be necessary to notify the appropriate utilities companies of a need for water, phone, and heat if there is economic hardship.

General Nursing and Treatment Orders

1. OB care provider refers client to perinatal home care program.

2. A plan of care is established between OB care provider, client, nurse, and insurer if indicated.

3. The clinical administrator will assign a perinatal nurse to complete an initial evaluation visit. The prenatal evaluation visit will include:

    a. Physical and psychosocial assessment using the Prenatal Universal Home Risk Assessment tool

    b. Classification of placenta previa

        1) Total: The placenta completely covers the internal cervical os

        2) Partial: The placenta partially covers the internal cervical os

        3) Low implantation of placenta: The placenta encroaches on the region of the internal cervical os and can be palpated on digital exploration about the cervix but does not extend beyond the margin of the internal os.

    c. When the initial bleeding started and how much painless bleeding occurred (usually bleeding will reoccur within hours or days after initial bleeding episode)

    d. Diagnostic data (hemoglobin, hematocrit, fibrinogen, coagulation studies)

    e. Biophysical assessment

      1) Position and presentation of fetus

      2) Presence or absence of uterine contraction (tocolytics)

      3) Baseline vital signs: temperature, pulse, respiration, blood pressure, and fetal heart rate

   f. Socioeconomic evaluation

      1) Determine whether home health aide services are required.

   g. Appropriate identifying information

      1) Client's name, address, and phone number

      2) Referring obstetrician, address, and phone number

      3) Insurance type and number

      4) Known drug allergies

      5) Type of home care, visits, and frequency

   h. Supplies and equipment needed

   i. Establishing plan of care, with short-term and long-term goals

4. Perinatal nursing visit

   a. Daily visits may be necessary during the first week, then evaluation by nurse and obstetrician weekly. This will be better determined after the initial nursing visit and completion of the Prenatal Universal Home Risk Assessment tool.

   b. A total nursing physical assessment is done with each visit.

      1) Cardiovascular: Assess for signs of hypotension, tachycardia, orthostatic hypotension, faint pulse rate.

      2) Respiratory: Assess breath sounds in all lung fields for any congestion or abnormal breath sounds; assess rate and lung expansion.

      3) Musculoskeletal: To maintain client on bed rest with bathroom privileges; maintain muscle tone by providing passive range-of-motion exercises.

      4) Metabolic: Monitor client's hemoglobin, hematocrit.

      5) Reproductive: Monitor contractions, bleeding, and fetal heart tones if any increase in contractions. Teach uterine self-palpation and how to maintain record of fetal movement, bleeding, or increase or decrease in fetal heart tones. Beyond normal limits, OB care provider must be called; obtain from OB care provider results from serial ultrasounds, NST, and challenge stress test. Obtain information on type of previa the client has.

        (a) Type I: Low placental implantation; lower edge of placenta does not cover the internal cervical os

        (b) Type II: Low placental implantation; the edge reaches the internal cervical os but does not cover it (marginal placenta previa)

      (c) Type III: The placenta completely covers the undilated cervix and only covers the internal os partially when cervix is dilated (partial placental previa)

      (d) Type IV: The placenta covers the internal cervical os when cervix is dilated or closed (complete placenta previa)

          NOTE: Placenta previa is three times more frequent after the age of 35 years. Prior uterine surgery or scar has also been shown to increase risk.

  6) Psychological: Educate client about her diagnosis and maintain physiologic and psychological homeostasis. Provide support and positive reinforcement to client and family members.

  7) Neurologic: Assess for signs of dizziness, blurred vision, general malaise, and headaches.

c. OB care provider update

  1) Update with OB care provider on a weekly basis.

  2) Review diagnostic data with OB care provider.

  3) Thirty-day review of plan of treatment.

Nursing Assessment

1. Activity

  a. Bed rest with or without bathroom privileges

  b. Physical activity should be restricted

  c. No vaginal examinations

  d. Douching is contraindicated

  e. Bathroom privileges

2. Diet

  a. Nutritional teaching

  b. High in fiber and increase in fluids because of increase in mobility

3. Education

  a. Placenta Previa

    1) Define diagnosis to client and client's family.

    2) Explain possible complications.

      (a) Hemorrhagic shock

      (b) Prematurity

    3) Emergency ambulance number by the phone

    4) Review signs and symptoms of placenta previa.

      (a) Bleeding may be slight or profuse.

      (b) Painless bright red bleeding

      (c) Signs of rigidity in abdomen

    5) Teach client signs and symptoms of adverse reactions to tocolytics.

    6) Educate client about premature labor and premature delivery.

  b. Childbirth education

    1) Teaching breathing and relaxation exercises

    2) Preparing client for possible Cesarean delivery

  c. Uterine monitoring system, if used

    1) Before or at time of first visit, uterine monitoring system is placed in client's home.

    2) Review of monitoring uterine contractions every visit

    3) Document the number of contractions at each monitoring interval on nursing clinical record. If there is an increase in contractions noted, then clarify what client was doing before medication and whether client still feels an increase in contractions.

    4) Notify OB care provider if monitoring system shows more than five contractions in 1 hour.

  d. Psychological Support

    1) Explain during each nursing visit all the procedures and answer any questions.

    2) Provide educational materials about premature infant.

    3) Perinatal support group

    4) Positive reinforcement and support

    5) Prepare client and family members for childbirth.

4. Medication

  a. Educate client about the actions and side effects of each medication.

  b. Review proper administration of medication during each nursing visit.

  c. Review any new medications that client might be receiving for any contraindications.

5. Follow-up Care

  a. Establish with client that, after delivery, a follow-up appointment with her health care provider is necessary for her and her baby.

  b. Encourage client to establish a yearly appointment with her OB care provider.

6. Individualized Treatment Plan

  a. Level I: Preventive

    1) Nursing visits: Weekly visits; can be decreased to once every other week

    2) Home health aide: 3 to 5 days per week

  b. Level II: Intermediate

    1) Nursing visits: 2 to 3 times per week for first 2 to 3 weeks, then decreasing to once per week

2) Home health aide: 3 to 5 days per week

c. Level III: Acute

    1) Nursing visits: Daily visits starting day of referral. Weekly reports to OB care provider, or if there is a problem, more frequently. Maintain bed rest; prepare for premature labor, delivery, or possibly premature baby; introduce childbirth education.

    2) Home health aide: 5 to 7 days per week

■ PERINATAL HOME CARE PROTOCOL FOR HYPEREMESIS GRAVIDARUM

Eligibility

1. Severe nausea and vomiting

2. Nutritional deficiency

3. Weight loss

4. Absence of severe dehydration and electrolyte imbalance

5. IV therapy at home

6. Assessment of risk using Prenatal Data Collection and Risk Scoring Tool

General Nursing and Treatment Orders

1. At the time of referral by the OB care provider, the following information is obtained:
   a. Client's name, address, and phone number
   b. Referring physician, address, and phone number
   c. Insurance type and number
   d. Known drug allergies
   e. Any medication client is taking
   f. Socioeconomic status of client
   g. Client's location—hospital or home
   h. Medical and obstetric history
   i. Laboratory values
   j. IV fluid orders

2. Perinatal nursing visit
   a. The clinical administrator will assign a perinatal nurse to make the initial evaluation visit using the Prenatal Universal Home Risk Assessment tool.
      1) Complete physical assessment:
         (a) Cardiovascular: Assess blood pressure and heart rate; hypotension may occur.
         (b) Respiratory: Auscultate lungs; be aware of deep, rapid breathing, depressed respiration, and shortness of breath on exertion.
         (c) Musculoskeletal: Assess for muscle cramping, tetany, hypotonicity, weakness, and tingling of ends of fingers.
         (d) Gastrointestinal: Assess for nausea, vomiting, cramping, diarrhea, weight loss, anorexia, gaseous distention of intestine, and silent intestinal ileus.

> (e) Genitourinary: Assess urine output (amount and concentration); check for ketones in urine.
>
> (f) Neurologic: Assess for disorientation, hyperactive deep reflexes, tremor, convulsions.
>
> (g) Reproductive: Assess uterine cramping, vaginal bleeding, and fetal heart rate if more than 12 weeks' gestation. Teach client uterine self-palpation and fetal movement counting if pregnancy has advanced to this point; most hyperemesis occurs before the client is able to assess these indicators.
>
> (h) Metabolic: Record temperature.
>
> (i) Skin: Assess skin turgor and color, tongue, and mucous membranes.
>
> (j) Psychological: Assess client's emotional status, encourage client to express concerns and problems related to pregnancy complications.

b. Intravenous therapy

1) Insert IV catheter and change every 72 hours if peripheral.
2) Examination of IV insertion site
3) Monitoring of intake and output
4) Drawing of blood for laboratory studies as ordered

c. OB care provider

1) The perinatal nurse will communicate daily with the OB care provider to review laboratory values, obtain IV orders, and report client status.

Nursing Assessment

1. Activity
   a. Ambulation as tolerated
   b. May require assistance because of muscle weakness

2. Diet
   a. Usually nulla per os (nothing by mouth; NPO) for 48 hours
   b. Once vomiting stops, oral fluids are introduced with gradual dietary progression as tolerated.

3. Education
   a. Educate client and family regarding:
      1) Infusion pump—settings, alarms, and when to call nurse
      2) Changing solution bags
      3) Assessing IV site for signs of infection, infiltration, phlebitis
   b. Teach client and family how to record intake and output.
   c. Instruct client in gradual reintroduction of fluids and food.

4. Medication

    a. Educate client on dose, frequency of administration, action, and side effects of any prescribed medication. Daily nurse visits should occur while client is receiving IV therapy, and nurse should be available on call 24 hours per day.

5. Psychological support

    a. Reassure client that her condition will improve.

    b. Evaluate family situation and provide emotional support.

    c. Assure client that a nurse is available 24 hours per day.

    d. Allow client and family to express concerns and problems.

▧ PERINATAL HOME CARE PROTOCOL FOR INTRAVENOUS FLUID ADMINISTRATION OF TOTAL PARENTERAL NUTRITION (TPN) AND INTRALIPIDS

Eligibility

1. Initial acute treatment completed, including diagnostic and surgical procedures as indicated

2. Laboratory values within normal range

3. Hickman catheter, central line has been placed.

4. Free of infection

5. Client demonstrates ability to cope with therapy.

6. Client and family have received instruction to recognize or prevent complications of therapy.

7. Preliminary risk assessed using the Prenatal Data Collection and Risk Scoring Tool.

Once a client has been identified as a high risk, the proper equipment and supplies must be ordered. The appropriate utilities companies must be notified of the need for water, phone, electricity, and heat if there is an economic hardship. Also, a plan for emergency transportation must be in place.

General Nursing and Treatment Orders

1. Before discharge
   a. The OB care provider refers the client to the perinatal home care program.
   b. The clinical administrator will assign a perinatal nurse to provide an initial evaluation visit to include:
      1) Physical and psychological assessment using the Prenatal Universal Home Risk Assessment tool
      2) The clinical administrator will assist in coordinating delivery of all pharmacy supplies and any other supplies from the medical supplier.
   c. Obtain laboratory test results, complete physical assessment, and pertinent past and current medical history from OB care provider.
      1) Appropriate identifying information:
         (a) Client's name, address, and phone number
         (b) Referring physician's name, address, and phone number

(c) Insurance types and numbers

(d) Known drug allergies

(e) Type of home care, visits, and frequency

(f) Medication and dietary treatment orders

(g) Supplies and equipment needed

(h) Evaluation of initial visit, establishing long-term and short-term goals.

(i) Perinatal nurse will sign and date Prenatal Universal Home Risk Assessment tool on day service is rendered.

(j) Notify electric company of medical priority concerning medical electrical equipment in case of power outage.

2. Perinatal nurse visit

   a. The nurse will perform physical assessment and examination to evaluate the following:

   1) Cardiovascular: Assess heart rate, rhythm, and presence of murmur. Palpate peripheral pulses and observe for edema.

   2) Respiratory: Auscultate breath sounds; note presence of rales as a sign of fluid overload. Observe rate, rhythm, and character of respiratory effort.

   3) Musculoskeletal: Assess muscle tone, vigor activity, movement of all extremities.

   4) Gastrointestinal: Check weight; auscultate bowel sounds. Determine frequency of stool.

   5) Genitourinary: Assess intake and output, color, smell of urine. Check urine for glucose or protein.

   6) Neurologic: Assess for neurologic deficit, orientation to time, place, person, irritability, level of consciousness.

   7) Reproductive: Assess for uterine contractions and irritability. Teach client uterine self-palpation and how to maintain record of fetal movement counts if appropriate, because many clients requiring this therapy are in their first trimester, and thus the pregnancy may not have progressed to the point yet where this is possible.

   8) Metabolic: Note temperature; assess for diaphoresis, clammy, cold skin, or skin that is warm to the touch. Check dextrostix.

   9) Psychological: Encourage and support client and family. Observe family interactions and verbalizations. Assess for need of community support.

10) Central line: Assess site of erythema, warmth, edema, drainage. Dressing must be changed using sterile technique every 48 hours or as ordered. Check flow rate of hyperalimentation and intralipids; adjust rate as indicated. Hang new fluids every 24 hours; to infuse either:

    (a) Over 24 hours or

    (b) Over 12 hours

       as determined by OB care provider and individual client's age and condition.

Nursing Assessment

1. Activity

    a. Activity limited, as tolerated

    b. Avoid activity that would risk dislodging catheter or disconnecting tubing.

2. Diet

    a. Nutritional requirements

       1) The average energy requirements for pregnant women according to age are

          (a) 11 to 14 years—2,500 calories daily

          (b) 15 to 18 years—2,400 calories daily

          (c) Over 19 years—2,400 calories daily

       2) Amino acid requirements for the same groups are

          (a) 11 to 14 years—76 g

          (b) 15 to 18 years—76 g

          (c) Over 19 years—74 g

       3) When calculating calorie intake, use one of the following methods:

          (a) 1 g dextrose = 3.4 kcal

          (b) 100 mL/kg $D_{10}W$ = 34 kcal/kg

          (c) 100 mL/kg $D_{30}W$ = 102 kcal/kg

          (d) Dextrose load (mg/kg/min)

          (e) g dextrose/day × 1,000 /weight (kg) over 1,440

       4) Lipids

          (a) One g/day liquid emulsions per 100 kcal is sufficient to prevent EFA (essential fatty acid) deficiency; however, additional fat emulsions are used generally to increase nonprotein calories.

          (b) Maximum intake: 3 g/kg/day

          (c) Available forms: 10% or 20% concentrations

          (d) The 20% concentration may result in lower plasma levels of triglyceride and cholesterol.

    b. Maintaining healthy diet

      1) If not NPO, determine intake type and amount as well as frequency.

      2) Review the food pyramid and the importance of balanced eating.

3. Medication

    a. Educate client on signs and symptoms of adverse reaction to any prescribed medication.

    b. Review any drug allergies.

4. Education

    a. Provide written instructions to client based on individual need.

    b. Provide teaching in prescribed procedure or treatment.

      1) Aseptic technique

      2) Catheter care

      3) Dressing changes

      4) Capping of catheter when not in use

      5) Handling and storage of parenteral nutrition solutions and tubing

      6) Preparing TPN infusion systems

      7) Attachment of infusion system to catheter

      8) How to infuse the correct solution at the correct rate

      9) Proper disposal of equipment, solutions, and sharps

    c. Safety

      1) Review home safety; identify and correct hazards in the home.

      2) Review signs of infection and intolerance to food.

      3) Stress importance of follow-up care.

    d. Intravenous site care

      1) Avoid bumping or other abuse at site.

      2) Review signs of infiltration and phlebitis and measures to be taken.

      3) Keep site clean and dry.

    e. Urine monitoring

      1) Educate client and family in method of daily dipsticking of urine for glucose or protein as ordered.

      2) Instruct client and family on maintaining accurate intake and output sheet.

5. Individualized treatment plan

    a. For client on 24-hour therapy:

      1) RN evaluation visit

      2) RN visit daily to remove outdated fluids and hang new fluids; and to change dressing

      3) Obtain weight.

    4) Measure intake, output, and urine monitoring.

    5) Provide comprehensive physical and psychosocial plan.

  b. For client on 12-hour therapy:

    1. RN evaluation visit

    2. RN visit twice per day to hang fluids and then to discontinue fluids; and to change dressing

    3. Obtain weight.

    4. Measure intake, output, and assess urine monitoring.

6. Individualized Treatment Plan Example:

Client name: _______________________   **Doctor name:** _______________________

Diagnosis: Intravenous fluid administration of hyperalimentation and intralipids

Equipment Order: Hyperal and intralipids—new setups B-D caps; alcohol swabs; Betadine ointment or solution; sterile gloves; masks; sterile 4×4s; bioclusive dressing; heparinized sodium for flush; 3-cc syringes; IV pole; infusion pump (2); Burretral chamber; tubing for appropriate pump; filters; 30″ extension tubing; three-way stopcocks; urine dipstix; lancets; dextrostix; needle disposal receptacle, other equipment as indicated by the pharmacy and medical supplier, intake/output sheets regularly used by the home health provider.

Laboratory test order: Electrolytes; triglycerides; cholesterol; liver function; calcium; phosphorus; magnesium; creatinine; BUN; total protein/albumin.

Diet Order:

Activity Order: ____

RN to phone Dr. _______________________ every _____________ days/week with patient report or update or immediately with any deviation from standard.

NURSING CARE PLAN: Diabetes Mellitus

CLIENT ASSESSMENT

Nursing History	Physical Examination	Diagnostic Studies	Third Trimester— Fetal Assessment

1. Complete assessment: client and family
2. Identification of client's predisposition to diabetes
  a. Recurrent pregnancy-induced hypertension (PIH)
  b. Previous large gestational age infants (~ 4,000 g)
  c. Hydramnios
  d. Unexplained fetal death
  e. Obesity
  f. Family history of diabetes
	1. Length of gestation
	2. Complaints of thirst and hunger
	3. Recurrent monilial vaginitis or urinary tract infection (UTI)
	4. Frequent urination beyond first trimester and before third trimester
	5. Fundal height greater than expected for gestation
	6. Obesity
	7. Funduscopic examination to detect any vascular changes
		1. Fasting plasma glucose (FPG)
		2. 3-hour GTT
		3. Urine test for glucose, ketones
		4. Ultrasound to evaluate fetal growth and detect hydramnios
		5. If woman has insulin-dependent diabetes mellitus (IDDM), glycosylated hemoglobin level (HbA_{1c}) determined
		6. Serum fructosamine screening is now used in some centers
		7. Maternal serum alpha-fetoprotein (AFP) screening
			1. Serial non-stress tests (NSTs)
			2. CST as necessary
			3. Serial ultrasound
			4. Biophysical profile to determine fetal maturity
			5. Amniocentesis and L/S ratio as necessary

Nursing Diagnosis	Nursing Interventions	Rationale	Evaluation
Altered nutrition: Potential for more than body requirements related to imbalance between intake and available insulin	Discuss importance of strict dietary control. Work with nutritionist and client to plan an individualized diet.	Dietary management is designed to ensure optimum fetal growth and normalize blood glucose levels. The greatest success occurs when a dietary plan is individualized to meet client needs and preferences.	Client understands her prescribed diet, follows it carefully, and gains the optimum amount of weight for her prepregnant size.

Client Goal: The client will understand and follow her prescribed diet as evidenced by weight gain within desired range, ability to discuss diet and plan menus, glycosylated hemoglobin (HbA_{1c}) levels in normal range.	Recommended intake: 30–35% kcal/kg body weight
	  12–20% protein
	  50–60% carbohydrate
	  20–30% fat
	Sodium intake may be restricted somewhat
		Recommended intake is designed to permit the following weight gain (Kitzmiller 1988):
		  Underweight 30′ lb
		  Desirable weight 24–30 lb
		  Overweight 20–24 lb
		  Very overweight 15–20 lb	

Rick for Injury: Related to possible complications secondary to hypoglycemia or hyperglycemia	Determine insulin needs: 1. Check lab results of FPG and 2-hour postprandial. 2. Test blood four times daily using Dextrostix.	Sufficient insulin must be present to enable proper carbohydrate metabolism to take place; pregnancy rquires a marked increase in circulating insulin to maintain normal blood glucose.	Client avoids episodes of hyperglycemia or hypoglycemia, or, if they occur, they are detected early and treated successfully. Insulin requirements become stabilized.

NURSING CARE PLAN: Diabetes Mellitus (Continued)

Nursing Diagnosis	Nursing Interventions	Rationale	Evaluation
Client Goal: Client will avoid injury associated with hypoglycemia or hyperglycemia as evidenced by absence of signs or symptoms, blood glucose readings in normal range, and stabilization of insulin requirements.	Teach use of home blood glucose monitoring device; determine amount of insulin based on sliding scale. Administer regular or NPH insulin, or combination, as ordered.	Fasting glucose level tends to be lower than nonpregnant value. Effectiveness of insulin may be reduced by presence of hPL.	
	Teach early signs of hypoglycemia; including sweating; periodic tingling; disorientation; shakiness; pallor; clammy skin; irritability; hunger; headache; blurred vision; and, if untreated, coma or convulsions.	Insulin requirements fluctuate widely during pregnancy because of factors mentioned in the text and because of lowered glucose tolerance, especially in the second half of pregnancy, and fluctuate during the intrapartal period because of depletion of glycogen stores during labor; fluctuations during puerperium are the result of an involuntary process; in addition, conversion of blood glucose into lactose during lactation may cause marked changes in glucose tolerance or hypoglycemia. Client needs to understand appropriate interventions because self-care at home in the event of hypoglycemia may save her life. Rapid treatment of hypoglycemia is essential to prevent brain damage because the brain requires glucose to function (skeletal and heart muscle can derive energy from ketones and free fatty acids).	

(continued)

NURSING CARE PLAN: Diabetes Mellitus (Continued)

Nursing Diagnosis	Nursing Interventions	Rationale	Evaluation
	Treat within minutes of onset:		
	a. Obtain immediate blood glucose level. If , 60 mg/dL, have client drink 8 oz milk (some agencies prefer to use ½ glass orange juice) and notify physican	Provides baseline information on glucose levels. Liquids are absorbed from the GI tract faster than solids.	
	b. If client is not alert enough to swallow, give 1 mg glucagon subcutaneously or intramuscularly; notify physician.	Glucagon triggers the conversion of glycogen stored in the liver to glucose.	
	c. If client is in labor with intravenous lines in place, 10–20 mL of 50% dextrose may be given IV.		
	Standing order should be available; notify physician.		
	Teach client early signs of hyperglycemia and treatment.	Client can recognize signs and administer self-treatment. Client also can report any symptoms that may occur.	
	Observe for signs of hyperglycemia such as polyuria, polydipsia, dry mouth, increased appetite, fatigue, nausea, hot flushed skin, rapid deep breathing, abdominal cramps, acetone breath, headache, drowsiness, depressed reflexes, oliguria or anuria, stupor, coma.		

NURSING CARE PLAN: Diabetes Mellitus (Continued)

Nursing Diagnosis	Nursing Interventions	Rationale	Evaluation
	Administer treatment; notify physician.	Administer insulin to restore body's normal metabolism of carbohydrate, protein, and fat.	
	a. Obtain frequent measurement of blood glucose; measure urine acetone.	Need to establish a baseline and to determine additional insulin dosage and prevent overtreatment; urine acetone indicates development of ketoacidosis.	
	b. Administer prescribed amount of regular insulin subcutaneously or intravenously, or combination of routes.	Regular insulin is used because it acts immediately and is of short duration.	
	c. Replace fluids IV, orally, or both.	Fluids are depleted in the process of ketoacidosis; hypotension can result from decreased blood volume due to dehydration.	
	d. Measure intake and output.	Polyuria is an early sign of hyperglycemia; oliguria develops with hypotension and decreased blood flow to the kidneys.	
	e. Observe for symptoms of circulatory collapse; monitor blood pressure and pulse.	Circulatory collapse can result from hypotension.	
Risk for Injury related to signs of UTI secondary to glycosuria.	Review preventive measures such as voiding frequently, voiding after intercourse, wiping from front to back, wearing cotton crotch underpants, drinking cranberry juice.	Preventive measures are designed to remove bacteria from the bladder, avoid contamination from the rectal area or outside sources, facilitate air flow in the perineal area, and acidify urine.	Client implements self-care measure to avoid UTI. If UTI develops, treatment is effective, and complications are avoided.

(continued)

NURSING CARE PLAN: Diabetes Mellitus (Continued)

Nursing Diagnosis	Nursing Interventions	Rationale	Evaluation
Client Goal: Client will be able to identify signs of developing UTI and appropriate self-care measures to help prevent UTI. If signs of UTI do develop, therapy will be effective in preventing injury from complications.	Teach signs of developing UTI, including urgency, frequency, dysuria, and hematuria; low back pain with kidney involvement. Obtain clean-catch urine for culture and sensitivity.	Incidence of UTI is increased in diabetes, possibly because the existence of glycosuria provides a rich medium for bacterial growth.	
	Administer prescribed antibiotics.	Antibiotic prescribed is specific to causative organism.	
	Encourage fluids to 2000–3000 mL/day. Measure intake and output.	Increased fluid intake promotes urinary removal of organisms.	
Knowledge deficit related to the disease, its treatment, its implications for the woman, her unborn child, and the birth process.	Provide teaching as indicated based on individualized assessment of couple's knowledge level: 1. Explain procedures 2. Allow them to ask questions	Decreasing fear and increasing knowledge will make the client a more effective member of the antepartal health team. Anticipatory guidance helps the couple prepare for the upcoming experience.	Client is able to discuss her condition and its implications, follows the recommendations of her caregivers, and correctly carries out self-care activities related to her diabetes.
Client Goal: Client and her partner will understand diabetes and its possible implications for her pregnancy as evidenced by their ability to administer insulin, to identify signs of hypo- or hyperglycemia, and to discuss basic information about birth and anticipated therapy measures.	3. Develop a teaching plan to discuss and provide opportunities to practice administering insulin. Provide written information. Include partner so he can administer insulin if necessary. 4. Assess their level of knowledge of childbirth and use this to teach about what is happening. 5. Provide information about possible changes to expect during labor and birth due to DM. Explain about IV insulin; continue monitoring of fetal status. Stress unchanged aspects of the experience.		

NURSING CARE PLAN: Diabetes Mellitus (Continued)

Nursing Diagnosis	Nursing Interventions	Rationale	Evaluation
Risk for Injury to fetus related to the effects of diabetes on uteroplacental functioning and fetal growth *Client Goal:* Client will be able to discuss rationale for fetal monitoring and testing, and will cooperate with fetal testing and assessment schedule.	Explain purpose of all tests and procedures: 1. Ultrasound as ordered to provide periodic assessment of fetal size 2. Fetal activity diary 3. Serial NSTs 4. CST if indicated 5. Measurement of lecithin/ sphingomyelin ratio and phosphatidyl glycerol levels to determine fetal lung maturity 6. Biophysical profile	Compliance is increased when client understands purpose of tests. Information about fetal growth and activity helps caregivers evaluate placental functioning, anticipate the need for cesarean birth, determine fetal maturity, and decide on best time for birth.	Client cooperates with fetal testing schedule. Fetus responds well to tests and shows evidence of normal growth and placental functioning.
Altered Family Processes related to client's diabetes mellitus (DM) and the need for hospitalization *Client Goal:* Family will deal successfully with the client's illness; plan for changes necessary after discharge; and share their thoughts, feelings, and concerns with each other.	Encourage visits from family members and older siblings. Discuss with client and family changes that are necessary after discharge with regard to insulin, diet, exercise, and so forth. Assist family to make specific plans. Arrange for social services to visit or for homemaker assistance if necessary after discharge. Give family members information about the frustration that can occur when a family member is ill. Provide opportunities for them to discuss their feelings. Offer suggestions for coping.	Illness in one family member impacts the entire family. Sometimes outside support is necessary to help the family deal with feelings and identify ways of dealing with the illness of a member.	Client and family cope successfully with illness, make necessary plans for managing after discharge, and discuss their feelings in an open, caring way.

Perinatal and Fetal Evaluation Training Program

Over the past decade, there has been a rapid expansion in the technology available for the care of clients during pregnancy. Over the same period, it has been recognized that, provided proper assessments are made, there are a number of clinical management techniques that will help to decrease fetal morbidity and mortality. For this reason, each home care visit involves the assessment of two clients: the mother and her fetus.

Assessment of the fetus begins with a history of family health, genetic history, determination of intrauterine environment based on the mother's physical and mental health, medications she takes, and her socioeconomic characteristics. The goal of fetal assessment is to diagnose intrauterine pathology, intervene when possible, and to prevent a calamitous event. Observations for genetic abnormalities, monitoring physical growth of the fetus, which reflects intrauterine nutrition and oxygenation, and documentation of the fetal ability to adapt to extrauterine life are all factors the perinatologist, obstetric (OB) care providers, and perinatal nurse evaluate.

Only the highest risk pregnancy will require home non-stress testing. Monitoring through home fetal evaluation at each nursing visit will allow proper documentation of normal fetal well-being. The antepartum home visits will help the mother focus on her developing infant as a person distinct from herself.

IDENTIFICATION OF HIGH RISK PREGNANCY

1. Diagnosis and pathophysiologic process
   a. Hypertension
   b. Intrauterine growth retardation (IUGR)
   c. Diabetes
   d. Premature labor (history of or presently arrested)
   e. Collagen vascular disease
   f. Coagulopathy—anticardiolipid antibody
   g. Heart and renal disease
   h. Rh—isoimmunization
   i. Abnormal placental function
      1) Placental infarction
      2) Placenta previa
      3) Placental abruption
   j. Fetal malformation
   k. Oligohydramnios

METHODS OF FETAL ASSESSMENT

1. Complete physical assessment
   a. Cardiovascular: Assess blood pressure and apical heart rate; hypotension may occur.
   b. Respiratory: Auscultate lungs bilaterally and respiratory rate; be aware of deep, rapid breathing, depressed respiration, and shortness of breath or exertion.
   c. Metabolic: Record temperature.
   d. Gastrointestinal: Assess nutritional status, weight, bowel sounds; assess for nausea, vomiting, cramping, diarrhea.
   e. Genitourinary: Assess urine output; check for glucose, protein, ketones in urine; assess for burning, hematuria, and frequency on urination.
   f. Reproductive: Assess fetal heart rate (FHR) (120 to 160 beats/min); assess for abdominal rigidness or tenderness, palpate size and contour of abdomen, assess for contractions, uterine cramping, or vaginal bleeding.
   g. Musculoskeletal: Assess for muscle cramping, tetany, hypotonicity, weakness.

    h. Neurologic: Assess for disorientation, dizziness, headaches, or blurred vision; assess deep reflexes.

    i. Skin: Assess skin turgor and color, tongue and mucous membranes.

    j. Psychological: Evaluate home environment and support system; assess client's emotional status, encourage client to express concerns and problems related to pregnancy complications.

2. Laboratory values

    a. Anemia status (hemoglobin and hematocrit)

    b. Abnormal coagulation factors

    c. Abnormal glucose levels

    d. Maternal blood group immunization

    e. Toxoplasmosis

    f. White blood count

    g. 24-Hour urine for protein, creatinine, estriol

3. Antenatal testing that should be tracked through course of care

    a. Ultrasound results (level I or level II)

    b. Biophysical profile

    c. Doppler flow study

Assessment of Fetal Placental Function

NON-STRESS TEST (NST)   Antepartum fetal evaluation is an observation that the fetus is safe through recording accelerations of the FHR in response to fetal activity, uterine contractions, or external stimulation.

In late gestation, the healthy fetus exhibits an average of 34 accelerations above the baseline FHR each hour. These accelerations denote that there is an intact neurologic system operating on the fetal heart. Fetal hypoxia will disrupt this pathway. Fetal accelerations are associated with fetal movement more than 85% of the time, and more than 90% of gross movements are accompanied by acceleration. The accelerations may not be present during fetal sleep, which has been shown to be approximately 40 minutes long. The other causes for absence of FHR accelerations are central nervous system (CNS) depressants such as narcotics, phenobarbital, beta-blocker propranol, and chronic smoking.

The NST should in most cases take only 10 to 15 minutes. It virtually has no contraindications. The client may be seated in a reclining position and on her left side to prevent supine hypotension syndrome. The client's blood pressure and pulse should be recorded before the NST and repeated every 10 minutes during the procedure. The Doppler ultrasound transducer and the tocodynamometer are applied to detect FHR, uterine contractions, and fetal movement. An event marker is used by the client to establish when she feels fetal movement. A reactive test requires that at least two accelerations of the FHR of 15 beats/min amplitude and 15 seconds' duration be observed in 20 minutes of monitoring. If this criteria for reactivity is not met, then an additional 20 minutes of the NST will be performed, with the expectation that the lack of fetal activity is attributable to fetal sleeping. Some techniques such as manually stimulating the fetus and increasing fetal glucose levels by administering orange juice to the mother will induce fetal activity. If fetal activity still does not increase, a consulting perinatologist is to be notified. At that time, the perinatologist will interpret the NST and proceed to manage the nonreactivity of the NST.

Perinatal and Fetal Evaluation Training Program: Home NST

1. Goal

    a. To achieve competency in performing, interpreting, and evaluating fetal well-being through NST in the home environment.

2. Objectives

    a. To identify high-risk pregnancies where antepartum fetal evaluation is indicated

    b. To define NST and explain the pathophysiology behind the performance of this type of fetal evaluation

    c. To apply the principles of physiology to electronic fetal monitoring and use this knowledge in effective assessment and management of an antepartum client

    d. To identify normal and abnormal FHR patterns

    e. To be able to identify the most common diagnosis that would indicate the use of antepartum fetal evaluation

3. Course Description

    a. Four- to six-week training in an antenatal testing unit or, if this is not possible, 3 months one-on-one training with experienced perinatal nurse doing NSTs.

    b. Introduction to the use of the Doppler ultrasound transducer and tocodynamometer system

4. Course Evaluation

    a. Nursing skills will be evaluated at the end of the training program. Home care visits will be evaluated daily for the first 2 weeks after course completion. Evaluation will be conducted by clinical administrator or designee.

5. Course Requirements

    a. Two years in field of maternal-child nursing preferred

    b. One year obstetric nursing

    c. Registered Nurse license

    d. One year experience in home care

    e. Malpractice insurance

6. Course textbook

    a. *Maternity Nursing: Family, Newborn, and Women's Health Care*, 18th edition, by Sharon J.

Procedure 5-1: Management of Non-Stress Test (NST)

1. Client is scheduled by perinatal visiting nurse.
2. Obtain prenatal record (when available).
3. Explain the procedure to the client.
4. Place client in bed or chair in semi-Fowler's position.
5. Apply external fetal monitor.
6. Take and record maternal blood pressure on monitor tracing with client's name, date, and time.
7. Observe for fetal reactivity.

8. Notify client's OB provider of reactivity.

9. If test is nonreactive (no fetal movement) after 20 minutes, do one or more of the following: change patient's position, massage or shake mother's abdomen, have her drink a cup of juice.
10. If nonreactive after 40 to 60 minutes, notify patient's OB provider
11. Interpret test as follows or call OB provider for interpretation, depending on institutional policy:
    a. Reactive: A minimum of two fetal movements over 20 minutes associated with FHR acceleration of at least 15 beats/min, lasting at least 15 seconds
    b. Nonreactive: Fewer than two fetal movements associated with accelerations

3. To allay fear
4. To ensure comfort

5. To obtain monitor tracing.

7. If four fetal heart rate (FHR) accelerations of 15 beats above baseline occur within a 20-minute period, the test is reactive.
8. To stimulate fetus. Fetal sleep cycle may last 20 minutes.

10. OB provider will be called and further orders obtained.

Non-Stress Test Chart

Non-Stress Test: Reactive
    Repeat in 1 week or as ordered

Non-Stress Test: Nonreactive (20 min)
    Uterine & fetal stimulation

Non-Stress Test: Nonreactive (20 after stimulation)
    Notify OB provider

Non-Stress Test: Nonreactive (80 min)
    Place on lateral side
    Insert IV
    Administer tocolytic
    Administer oxygen
    If then reactive, repeat NST daily.
    If not reactive after these measures, call ambulance service and hospital.

(continued)

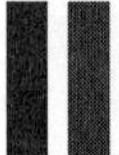

Procedure 5-1: Management of Non-Stress Test (NST) (Continued)

Description of NST Management Chart

NST is performed:

If Reactive
1. *Repeat test in 1 week*
2. *If nonreactive test becomes reactive after 80 minutes*
   a. *Repeat NST daily*

If Nonreactive
1. *If nonreactive after 20 minutes*
   a. *Provide uterine and fetal stimulation*
2. *If nonreactive after another 20 minutes*
   a. *Notify OB care provider*
3. *If nonreactive after 80 minutes*
   a. *Place patient on left side*
   b. *Insert IV*
   c. *Administer tocolytic medication*
   d. *Administer oxygen*
4. *If still nonreactive*
   a. *Notify ambulance*
   b. *Send to hospital*

Reeder, Leonide L. Martin, and Deborah Koniak-Griffin. Philadelphia: Lippincott-Raven Publishers, 1997.

   b. *Fetal Monitoring Interpretation*, by Micki Cabaniss. Philadelphia: JB Lippincott, 1993.

Management of Non-Stress Test

1. Purpose

   a. To evaluate fetal status through fetal heart activity and body motion assessment (see Procedure 5-1)

2. Objective

   a. Acceleration with fetal movement is indicative of fetal well-being.

3. Indications

   a. Diabetes

   b. Sickle cell disease

   c. Advanced maternal age

   d. Intrauterine growth retardation

   e. Hypertension

   f. Preeclampsia

   g. Post dates

   h. Previous stillbirth

    i. Maternal heart disease

    j. Decreased fetal movement

    k. RH-sensitized mother

    l. Previous neonatal demise

4. Equipment

    a. External fetal monitor—aquasonic

    b. Abdominal belts

    c. Tocodynamometer

    d. Phono/Ultrasound transducer

    e. Aquasonic gel

CHAPTER 6

Home Monitoring Program

■ PERINATAL HOME CARE PROGRAM

Uterine Monitoring

The purpose of home uterine activity monitoring is to prevent a premature birth by detecting the signs of preterm labor early, before labor is well established. Uterine activity monitoring can be conducted by either electronic monitoring or self-palpation. Electronic monitoring has proved beneficial in detecting both contractions and uterine irritability. When electronic monitors are not an option (not available, no insurance coverage), the client can perform self-palpation. Studies have shown that the ability of clients who use self-palpation to detect uterine activity varies for each individual. For either electronic monitoring or self-palpation, two 1-hour sessions should be conducted per day by the client: 1 hour during the most active time of the morning and 1 hour during the most active time during the evening.

ELECTRONIC MONITORING
To monitor contractions with an electronic monitor, the client should follow the instructions provided by the manufacturer. The nurse should review, reinforce, and determine the client's understanding of instructions. If the client detects four or more contractions per hour, she should call her OB care provider or follow the prescribed regimen for managing increased uterine activity.

SELF-PALPATION
For self-palpation, the client should:

1. Lie down with a pillow behind her back and tilt slightly to her left side.

2. Place her fingertips on the lower sides of her abdomen to feel for tightening of the entire uterine muscle, signifying a contraction.

3. Use her watch to time the length of the contraction as well as the time between each contraction.

Risk Factors That May Indicate Need for Home Uterine Monitoring

1. Hypertension
   a. Clients with a history of or current hypertension during pregnancy may be at increased risk for the development of preeclampsia and abnormal uteroplacental blood flow and function, with consequent fetal growth retardation and the risk of fetal hypoxia or asphyxia.

2. Intrauterine fetal growth retardation
   a. Clients with a history of or current fetal growth retardation are at increased risk for the development of fetal hypoxia and asphyxia, especially if the growth retardation is caused by abnormal placental transfer of oxygen and nutrients associated with drug use, hypertension, poor nutrition, preeclampsia, or poor uteroplacental function.

3. Premature labor or premature cervical dilation
   a. After appropriate treatment of premature labor or cervical dilation, once the process has arrested, the client remains at risk for recurrence of either labor or silent cervical dilation for the remainder of the pregnancy. Clients with multiple gestation, polyhydramnios, urinary tract infection, or sepsis are at increased risk.

4. Diabetes mellitus
   a. This disease poses a risk for abnormal maternal or fetal carbohydrate metabolism, as manifested by hyperglycemia or hypoglycemia, as well as a risk for abnormal fetal growth (either excessive or too little) and increases the risk for hypertensive complications of pregnancy.

5. Previous miscarriage
   a. These clients are at an increased risk for both recurrent miscarriage and premature delivery (caused by either premature labor or premature cervical dilation).

6. Collagen vascular disease
   a. This disease may affect both maternal and fetal (ie, placental) circulation, increasing the risk of uteroplacental insufficiency with consequent abnormal fetal growth and lack of well-being.

7. Maternal coagulopathy
   a. Especially when the mother carries a circulating anticoagulant (ie, anticardiolipid antibody or lupus anticoagulant), there is an extremely high risk of diminished circulation through the uterus and placenta and the development of placental infarctions, thereby increasing the risk of uteroplacental insufficiency with consequent fetal growth retardation, asphyxia, and possibly death.

8. Maternal cardiac disease

    a. With compromised cardiac reserve, both circulation and oxygenation to the pelvic area (including the uterus and fetus) may be diminished, thereby increasing the risk of uteroplacental insufficiency.

9. Maternal renal disease

    a. When maternal renal function is compromised to the point of a significant decrease in creatinine clearance and elevation of maternal serum creatinine and BUN, the risk of uteroplacental insufficiency and hypertensive complications are greatly increased.

10. Fetal anomaly

    a. Some fetal anomalies carry an increased risk of premature delivery (eg, when associated with hydramnios or multiple gestations) or abnormal fetal development and oxygenation (eg, some fetal cardiac anomalies).

11. Red blood cell isoimmunization

    a. Especially with Rh and anti-Kell disease, fetal hemolytic anemia may progress to the point of fetal hypoxia and asphyxia of fetal hydrops with associated hydramnios. These processes carry the risk of fetal death and premature delivery.

12. Abnormal placentation

    a. With placenta previa, abruptio placenta, or placental infarctions, abnormal transfer of oxygen and nutrients to the fetus increase the risk of growth retardation and chronic asphyxia, and the mother carries an increases risk of obstetric hemorrhage.

13. Multiple Gestation

    a. This carries an increased risk of premature delivery, abnormal fetal growth, abnormal placentation, gestational diabetes, hypertensive complications, fetal anomalies, and maternal anemia.

    Premature ruptured membranes or evidence of uterine infection (ie, chorioamnionitis) should almost always be treated in the hospital and thereby disqualifies most clients for home care. Certain exceptions (eg, very immature fetus) may be considered after perinatal consultation.

CHAPTER 7

Childbirth Education

Childbirth education is a crucial component in helping to promote a positive outcome for the woman and her newborn. Knowledge of the changes brought about by pregnancy can help reduce fear and anxiety and thus stress levels in the body. Knowledge of potential problems can result in timely, lifesaving interventions for the fetus and the mother. We live in a society in which the miracle of birth has been hidden away in the hospital and in some ways mysticized. Therefore we cannot assume that all women are well informed on the processes of pregnancy, childbirth, and parenting. All women should be afforded access to childbirth education. One of the most important roles of the perinatal nurse, no matter which clinical environment he or she works in, is to make sure this access is provided.

This chapter provides a three-class childbirth education program outlining the topics that should be incorporated into any childbirth education service. The classes may be offered in the traditional community setting (ie, the obstetric [OB] provider's office, hospital, church, and so forth) or, for those women whose complications of pregnancy require bed rest or activity limitations, may be provided in one-on-one in the client's home. Perinatal nurses using the class outlines of this chapter will find it helpful to copy the sections being taught for a specific client. Some helpful educational tools for clients are also located in Chapter 8. It is also recommended that the perinatal nurse obtain a current obstetric textbook for reference and develop a visual aids library, which might include videos and charts. Resources for these materials are noted within the chapter.

CLASS I

1. Introductions

    a. Childbirth educator

    b. Clients and coaches

    c. Class objectives and outline

        1) To educate on prenatal, perinatal, and postnatal facts and expected experiences so as to promote a safe, healthy delivery and future for mother and baby.

2. *Miracle of Life* (Recommended video, available through Nova, produced by the Corporation for the Public Broadcasting Service)

3. Maternal changes and discomforts during pregnancy

    a. Expected physical changes

        1) Reproductive

            (a) Uterine expansion from pear size to greater than size of baby permitted by expansion of actual size of uterine muscle cell

            (b) Cervix softens and a mucus plug forms in the cervical canal to prevent ascent of bacteria, which could cause infection.

            (c) Ovaries cease to produce eggs, but secrete hormones to assist with maintenance of pregnancy.

            (d) Changes occur in vaginal secretions that help prevent bacterial growth, but in turn allow overgrowth of normal yeast, which can lead to yeast infections. Normal vaginal secretions should be white and slightly thicker than usual. Menstrual cycles usually cease. Do not use douches without consulting with doctor (douches usually not recommended).

            (e) In the breasts, superficial veins become noticeable, nipples become more erect, areola darken, and colostrum may leak from nipples in third trimester.

        2) Respiratory

            (a) Tidal volume, the amount of air breathed with each respiration, increases throughout pregnancy.

            (b) Diaphragm is elevated because of the expanding uterus (chest will expand up to 6 cm to compensate for decreased breathing area so enough air can be inhaled).

        3) Cardiovascular

            (a) Blood volume and heart rate increase throughout pregnancy.

(b) Blood pressure decreases slightly during first two trimesters of pregnancy; increases in third trimester.

(c) Edema occurs because the growing uterus makes blood flow from extremities more difficult. There is a tendency for edema especially in the extremities (which can ache); blood stagnation; varicose veins, hemorrhoids; and postural hypotension (especially if lying on back and then rising quickly), which can make pregnant woman dizzy, clammy, and feel slightly faint. Therefore, she should rise slowly.

(d) Red blood cells (RBC) increase in number with pregnancy, but if amount of iron in blood (the part of blood that carries the oxygen to the cells) does not increase (because client does not take her prenatal vitamins and iron), then the needed increase of oxygen to tissues and the baby does not occur.

(e) White blood cells ([WBCs]infection fighters) increase in number.

(f) The substances that stop bleeding (otherwise known as blood clotting factors), increase in amount.

(g) There is an increased chance of a venous thrombosis (a blood clot) caused by edema, increased RBCs, WBCs, and clotting factors.

4) Gastrointestinal

(a) Nausea and vomiting are common in the first trimester. If client is vomiting more than once a day, she should notify her doctor. Certain smells and tastes may aggravate it, or reversely, mother may crave eating nonnutritive substances (called pica) such as clay, corn starch, or soap.

(b) Gum tissue may soften and bleed when brushing teeth.

(c) Increased saliva

(d) Heartburn is the reflux of gastric acid into the esophagus caused by softening of the sphincter between the esophagus and the stomach and pressure on the stomach from the uterus.

(e) Bloating and constipation occur because of the increased size of the uterus, displacement of intestines, and decreased gastric motility. The client should not use enemas or laxatives without consulting her OB care provider. Increase fluid and fiber to prevent constipation.

(f) Hemorrhoids occur as a result of constipation or decreased venous return (engorged veins).

(g) Gallstones may be a problem because of the client's disposition to decreased emptying of gallbladder from the pressure of the growing uterus.

5) Urinary

    (a) Bladder pressure from uterus increases chance of infection or trauma, and decreased retention capacity. It is normal to pass urine more frequently but urination should not be painful or burn.

6) Skin and Hair

    (a) The client may experience some or all of the following: increased pigment in areola, nipples, perineal area, midline; facial chloasma (mask of pregnancy), irregular pigmentation of cheeks, forehead, and nose.

    (b) Hyperactive sweat glands

    (c) Striae, or stretch marks, may be found on the abdomen, legs, or breasts.

    (d) Vascular spider nevi can be found on face, neck, arms, or legs. They usually resemble a spider and disappear after pregnancy.

    (e) Hair follicles may become dormant after stimulation of pregnancy, and the client may lose some hair, which will grow back.

7) Metabolism

    (a) Many women lose weight during the first trimester because of nausea, vomiting, and food intolerances, but should regain 16 to 30 lbs (OB care provider will recommend appropriate gain) in the last two trimesters.

    (b) Water retention is a normal occurrence because of numerous metabolic changes during pregnancy, and will be evidenced by increased voiding and edema).

8) Musculoskeletal

    (a) Sacral bones relax because of hormonal changes. This often causes a waddling gait with slight separation at symphysis pubis.

    (b) Some postural changes occur to compensate for weight shift. This is to maintain the body's center of gravity, but it also contributes to muscle aches. Caution: as pregnancy progresses, be aware that labor contractions can feel similar to back pain. Try to discern between the two by feeling abdomen for regular patterned movements or tightening of muscle and also wear flat shoes to decrease chance of falling.

9) Neurologic

    (a) Rest is very important, so get enough of it!!!!

    (b) DO NOT USE ANY MEDICATION (ORAL, TOPICAL, RECTAL, INHALANT, OR OTHERWISE) WITHOUT CONSULTING OB CARE PROVIDER—IT COULD HARM THE FETUS!

b. Special needs and concerns of mother

  1) Emotional: Mood swings, postpartum depression, support systems

2) Nutrition: Adequate amounts of many nutrients from the food pyramid are necessary to provide the building blocks for the new baby and to keep mom healthy

3) Dental Care: Get checkups to ensure good dental health and no infection

4) Avoid the following situations:

   (a) Drugs: Prescription, over-the-counter (unless approved by OB care provider), and street drugs should be avoided. All drugs pass to the fetus, and, although they may be safe for adults, their effect on the fetus is harmful or unknown.

   (b) Alcohol: No safe intake level is known, so abstaining from alcohol is encouraged. Alcohol has been proven to have effects on the baby.

   (c) Tobacco: Decreases oxygen to mom and baby and can decrease growth of baby. Ask OB provider about cessation classes.

   (d) Radiation: Always tell radiologist you are pregnant. X-rays that are not immediately necessary can be postponed.

5) Safer sex: Use of condoms during pregnancy to prevent infection is imperative. You can continue with normal sexual activity unless uncomfortable, painful, or OB care provider recommends against it.

6) Exercise: Maintain level of exercise accomplished in prepregnant state unless told by OB care provider that complications of pregnancy or medical problems limit activity; passive muscle tightening and relaxation, including Kegel exercises, should be performed.

7) Danger signs

   (a) Bleeding: Inform the OB provider about any amount of bleeding to determine if there is a problem.

   (b) Illness: Any fever, vomiting, diarrhea, headache, blurred vision, chills

   (c) Seizures are usually associated with eclampsia in pregnancy; preeclampsia, progression of proteinuria, hypertension (and increase in base pressure of more than 30/15 mmHg), and edema; eclampsia involves these symptoms accompanied by seizures.

   (d) Baby not moving around as usual: It is a good idea to monitor fetal movement regularly throughout day to get used to normal fetal activity to aid in awareness if a decrease in activity occurs (Client information available on page 95.) Fetal movements are detected by the mother on average around 16 weeks. Some women with first pregnancies may feel movement for several weeks without realizing it is the fetus (They may think it is gas.).

   (e) Strong feeling of "Something is not quite right"

   (f) Abnormal vaginal discharge: yellow, green, foul smelling, cheesy

    (g) Abdominal pain

    (h) Swelling of face or fingers

    (i) Severe headaches or blurring vision

c. Possible or actual signs and symptoms of impending labor:

1) Sudden burst of energy very soon before actual labor begins (nesting instinct)

2) Lightening: the feeling that the baby has dropped lower in abdomen

3) Discharge of pinkish mucous plug or unusual vaginal discharge

4) Rupture of amniotic membrane (water breaks as a trickle or gush): Note color and any odor of amniotic fluid if not in hospital. If you even suspect your water has broken, go to the hospital.

5) Abdominal cramping, vaginal, thigh, or back pain or pressure

6) Regular contractions with or without pain over more than 1 hour

    (a) Contractions: Monitor for length, regularity, and duration. Monitor by feeling abdomen with fingertips, feeling for tightening and loosening.

    (b) Timing contraction interval: Time from beginning of one contraction to the beginning of another contraction

    (c) Timing contraction duration: Time from beginning of contraction to end of contraction

d. Stages of labor: Breathing techniques (Detailed description is provided at the end of this chapter.)

1) Stage I: Dilation from 0 to 10 cm; three phases of Stage I

    (a) Early: Mild contractions, up to 5 cm dilation. Regular breathing to conserve energy with slow deep breath before and after each contraction. Coach should check for muscle tensing and do gentle massage if woman desires (with flat hand, center to outer body). Relaxation techniques also may be incorporated throughout labor.

    (b) Active: Moderate contractions, 5 to 8 cm dilation. Pick focal point, concentrate on it throughout contraction. Regular breathing increasing in speed, working into howt breathing as needed with the increase in pain (see Breathing Techniques below).

    (c) Panting: 10 cm dilation. Just as it sounds; pant as if out of breath. OB provider may request this to help control delivery.

        Practice: Caution—do not push for real when practicing!

2) Stage II: From 10 cm dilation to birth of baby.

    (a) Transition: Severe contractions, 8 to 10 cm dilation. Howt breathing to prevent hyperventilation during contraction.

(b) Pushing: With contractions, deep breath in and out before contraction; deep breath in and hold, bear down with bowel movement muscles for 10 seconds or as long as possible with the direction of the OB care provider during the contraction, then deep cleansing breath after push to oxygenate mother and baby.

Practice: Caution—do not push for real when practicing!

3) Stage III: From birth of baby to delivery of placenta

4. Embryonic/fetal growth and development

  a. Nagele's Rule: Take the first day of the last menstrual period, subtract 3 months, and add 7 days to determine estimated delivery date.

  b. Fetal growth chart handout: Use available materials, or see resources at the end of this chapter.

  c. Techniques to assess fetal growth and development

    1) Abdominal girth measurement: a good indicator between 13-28 weeks (Box 7-1)

    2) Ultrasound: not always done solely to determine sex of baby

      (a) Biparietal diameter (BPD)

      (b) Femur length (second to third trimester)

      (c) Abdominal circumference of fetus (most useful at 34 to 36 weeks): Use head circumference and abdominal circumference ratio to assess disproportion between head and body and to assess fetal weight.

5. Resources

  a. Prenatal care and childbirth education

  b. Medicaid/HMO/Commercial insurance

  c. Women, Infants and Children's Federal Nutrition Program (WIC), if eligible.

  d. Other

6. Labor

  a. True versus false: Labor is said to be true if it results in effacement and dilation

  b. Preterm labor: Before 37 weeks' gestation

    1) Newborn complications related to preterm birth

      (a) Respiratory difficulty and increased chronic respiratory problems

      (b) More prone to illnesses and feeding problems

      (c) In general, all organs have not fully matured. All bodily systems are not functioning as well as those of a full-term normal newborn, which subsequently causes the baby to have numerous problems, making the early months of life difficult.

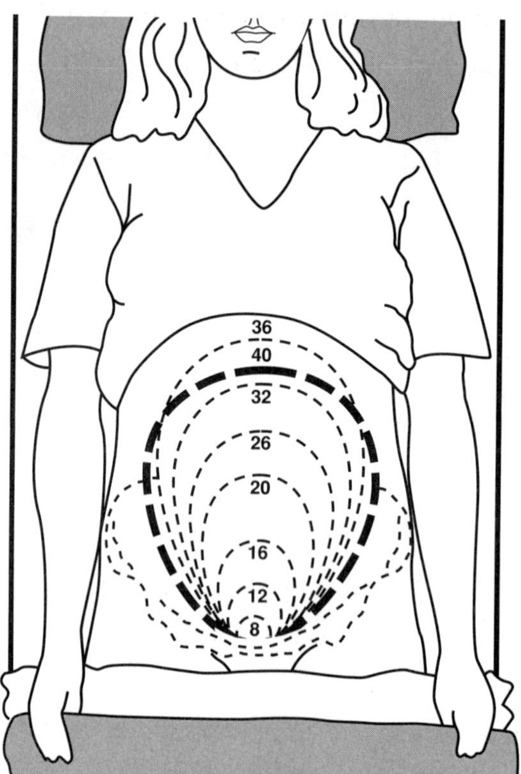

Fundal height is used as an indicator of fetal growth in relation to uterine size and weeks of gestation. McDonald's technique is to use pliable, not stretchable, paper tape to measure the distance from the upper border of the symphysis pubis to the top of the uterine fundus.

McDonald's Rule
   Height of fundus (cm) 2 2/7 4 gestation in lunar months.
   Height of fundus (cm) 2 8/7 4 gestation of pregnancy in weeks.

Considerations in using fundal height measurement: Factors such as hydramnios, multiple gestation, very large fetus, and obesity affect measurement accuracy. For women over 200 lbs., subtract 1 cm. from the measurement obtained. Approaches must be standardized when more than one caregiver is taking serial measurements.

2) Prevention

(a) Stop any smoking, intake of drugs and alcohol.

(b) Eat balanced, nutritious meals; gain appropriate weight.

(c) Signs of preterm labor: Any signs and symptoms of impending labor before 37 weeks

(d) Intervention: Empty bladder; lie down on left side at least 1 hour (increases oxygen to baby and uterus); drink at least 3 to 4 glasses of fluid while resting; feel abdomen and record pattern of contractions; if signs and symptoms do not cease, notify OB care provider with your name, due date, and signs and symptoms.

▊ CLASS II

1. Introductions
   a. Childbirth educator
   b. Clients and coaches
   c. Class content

2. Labor Discussion (Review)
   a. Contractions: Monitor for length, regularity, and duration. Monitor by feeling abdomen with fingertips, feeling for tightening and loosening.
      1) Timing contraction interval: Time from beginning of one contraction to the beginning of another contraction
      2) Timing contraction duration: Time from beginning of contraction to end of contraction
   b. True versus false labor: Labor is said to be true if it results in effacement and dilation.
   c. Premature: Before 37 weeks' gestation.
      1) Newborn complications related to preterm birth
         (a) Respiratory difficulty and increased chronic respiratory problems
         (b) More prone to illnesses; feeding problems
         (c) In general, all organs have not fully matured. All body systems are not functioning as well, which subsequently causes the baby to have numerous problems, making the early months of life difficult.
      2) Prevention
         (a) Stop any smoking, drugs, alcohol.
         (b) Eat balanced, nutritious meals; gain appropriate weight.
         (c) Signs of premature labor: Any signs or symptoms of impending labor before 37 weeks.
         (d) Intervention: Empty bladder; lie down on left side at least once per hour (increases oxygen to baby and uterus); drink at least 3 to 4 glasses of fluid while resting; feel abdomen and record pattern of contractions; if signs and symptoms do not cease, notify OB care provider with your name, due date, and signs and symptoms.

   d. Possible or actual signs and symptoms of impending labor

      1) Sudden burst of energy very soon before actual labor begins (nesting instinct)

      2) Lightening: the feeling that the baby has dropped lower in abdomen

      3) Discharge of pinkish mucous plug or unusual vaginal discharge

      4) Rupture of amniotic membrane (water breaks as a trickle or gush): Note color and any odor of amniotic fluid if not in hospital. If you even suspect your water has broken, go to the hospital.

      5) Abdominal cramping, vaginal, thigh, or back pain or pressure

      6) Regular contractions with or without pain for longer than 1 hour.

        (a) Contractions: Monitor for length, regularity, and duration. Monitor by feeling abdomen with fingertips, feeling for tightening and loosening.

        (b) Timing contraction interval: Time from beginning of one contraction to the beginning of another contraction

        (c) Timing contraction duration: Time from beginning of contraction to end of contraction

   e. Stages of labor: Breathing techniques (Detailed description is provided at the end of this chapter.)

      1) Stage I = dilation from 0 to 10 cm; three phases of Stage I

        (a) Early: Mild contraction , 0 to 5 cm dilation. Regular breathing to conserve energy with slow deep breath before/after each contraction. Coach should check for tense muscles and do gentle massage if woman desires (with flat hand—center to outer body). You can also incorporate any relaxation techniques which work for you throughout labor.

        (b) Active: Moderate contractions, 5 to 8 cm dilation. Pick focal point, concentrate on it throughout contraction, regular breathing increasing in speed, working into howt breathing as needed with the increase in pain.

        (c) Panting: 10 cm dilation Just as it sounds; pant as if out of breath. OB provider may request this to help control delivery.

          Practice: Caution—do not push for real when practicing!

      2) Stage II: From 10 cm dilatation to birth of baby

        (a) Pushing: With contractions and provider direction, push, breathing deep breath in and out before contraction, deep breath in and hold, bear down with BM muscles for 10 seconds or as long as you can with the direction of the OB provider during the contraction, then deep cleansing breath after push to oxygenate you and the baby.

          Practice: Caution—do not push for real when practicing!

      3) Stage III: From birth of baby to delivery of placenta

f. Labor and Delivery Videos

    1) Videos can be obtained through medical libraries and writing to childbirth education organizations such as Lamaze and International Childbirth Education Association for information. Some excellent films also can be found in or ordered by the local video store. Childbirth Graphics also offers some fine selections.

3. Special childbirth procedures and techniques

  a. Maternal monitoring

    1) Health history

    2) Vital signs

    3) Weight

    4) Lungs

    5) Heart

    6) Fundus: At 40 weeks should be at base of xiphoid process

    7) Edema: Swelling

    8) Energy: Conserve strength for labor

    9) Labor status: Dilation, effacement of cervix, length and duration of contractions, and evaluation of fetal heart tones

    10) Contractions assessed by:

      (a) Palpation: Hand placed on fundus to feel duration, frequency, and intensity

      (b) External uterine monitor: Indirect method to monitor frequency and duration (not intensity) by small pressure-sensitive disk held tight to the abdomen by a belt, recording increases and decreases in pressure from contractions.

      (c) Internal monitor: Pressure-sensitive catheter is inserted into uterus and assesses contraction frequency, duration, and intensity.

      (d) Dilation: Opening of cervix from 0 to 10 cm, assessed by vaginal examination

      (e) Effacement: Thinning and softening of cervix, assessed by vaginal examination

      (f) Fetal descent: Movement of baby down birth canal, assessed by vaginal examination

      (g) Membranes: Assess whether amniotic sac has ruptured. If unsure, can use nitrazine strips.

      (h) Psychological and emotional response to labor

  b. Fetal Monitoring

    1) Fetal heart rate (FHR): Normally 120 to 160 beats/min. If less or greater than this, could mean fetal distress

    2) Methods of assessing FHR

      (a) Fetoscope: type of stethoscope

    (b) Electronic fetal monitoring

    (c) External: An ultrasound transducer is placed on abdomen above gel substance that helps conduct sound. The results are printed on a continuous screen and graph paper.

    (d) Internal: A spiral electrode is attached to the fetus' scalp or buttocks, providing another continuous but clearer printout of FHR.

    (e) Presentation and position can be assessed by inspection, palpation, ultrasound of abdomen, and vaginal examination. This is important because it affects how well, if at all, fetus will pass through canal.

    (f) Activity

    (g) Fetal scalp stimulation test: Stimulate fetal scalp, through vaginal examination, to assess response in FHR.

    (h) Fetal scalp sampling is acquiring a scalp blood specimen to assess acid/base balance (acidity indicates fetal distress).

    (i) Percutaneous umbilical blood sampling is a sample of cord blood obtained through mother's abdomen.

c. Analgesia and Anesthesia

    Although analgesics and anesthetics affect the fetus, so do the pain and stress of labor. Analgesia will decrease the pain; anesthesia will completely block the pain. You should discuss pain relief with your clinician before the day of labor. Be sure to let your OB care provider know if pain relief is not working. You and your baby will be monitored throughout the time anesthesia/analgesia is used.

  1) Systemic drugs (usually given by intravenous route)

    (a) Narcotic analgesics: Demerol (meperidine)

    (b) Sedatives: barbiturates

  2) Regional analgesia and anesthesia: Affects a certain area; can be a single dose or continuous by indwelling catheter

    (a) Types of pain blocks

      (1) Lumbar epidural: This is given through injection into the spinal vertebrae in the epidural space. It affects the vagina and perineum, given in first and second stages of labor.

      (2) Pudendal: This is given through injection into the spinal vertebrae, hyperbaric subarachnoid. It affects the perineum and lower vagina, given in the second stage, and just before birth to provide anesthesia for episiotomy or low forceps delivery.

      (3) Local infiltration: This is given by injection into the perineum. It affects the

perineum and is administered just before birth to provide anesthesia for episiotomy.

3) General anesthesia

(a) May be needed for cesarean delivery or surgery because of complications or planned procedures

(b) Can be inhalation or intravenous or a combination of both

d. Delivery facilitation

1) Mechanical

(a) Forceps: Assist by providing traction to pull fetus, and a means to turn the head to the most agreeable position to come out

(b) Vacuum: A suction cup is applied to baby's head to assist its delivery.

(c) Both forceps and vacuum pulling are done during contraction to promote the quickest delivery.

(d) Episiotomy: To enlarge opening of perineum to facilitate birth. There are three types of incisions: midline, which is the quickest to heal; mediolateral, which provides the most space for exit but takes longer to heal; and tearing, a natural perineal skin tear.

2) Medicinal

(a) Pitocin: Increases strength of or induces uterine contractions; often results in stronger contractions, thus a "harder" labor

(b) Pitocin (oxytocin) also can be used when labor is not progressing as a result of slow dilation or ineffective contractions.

e. Cesarean Birth

1) Procedure

(a) During a planned cesarean delivery, patient and doctor should mutually agree on cesarean delivery well before due date if possible.

(b) Teaching of frequent turning, coughing, deep breathing, incision care, and splinting for postoperative period may be done.

(c) Woman can have nothing by mouth for a certain period before surgery.

(d) A urinary catheter will be inserted.

(e) Abdomen will be cleaned and sterilized.

(f) An IV line will be inserted, usually in an arm.

(g) Anesthesia and analgesia will be used; the type depends on many factors, such as whether the cesarean section was planned or an emergency (general anesthesia is usually used for emergencies).

(h) Every effort should be made to include the father in the birth experience if it is desired.

       (i) The cesarean is performed.

       (j) The baby is taken to warmer and assessed and cared for after bonding with mother if appropriate (mother is conscious).

      (k) Pitocin may be given to increase uterine contraction and decrease bleeding.

       (l) Mother will go to recovery room, where she will be closely monitored until she has recuperated from anesthesia.

     (m) Incision and fundus will be frequently checked.

     (n) Coughing and deep breathing should be done about every 2 hours.

     (o) The urine output in the catheter bag will be measured.

     (p) Postoperative pain relief should be provided.

2) Purpose or Cause

    (a) Done for many reasons: to facilitate a safer, quicker, or necessary method of birth

3) Vaginal birth after cesarean (VBAC)

    (a) Is possible, depending on the reason for the previous cesarean delivery and the type of incision

4) Complications related to cesarean delivery

    (a) Longer recovery period than vaginal birth

    (b) Possible complications related to surgery

5) Expected recovery

    (a) Follow recommendations from OB care provider related to activity, skin care, medications, and follow-up appointments.

4. Preparation for hospital stay

  a. Your hospital bag

    1) The average stay for an uncomplicated vaginal delivery is 24 to 48 hours, for a cesarean delivery, 3 to 4 days. The woman will need one to two nightgowns, underwear, a nursing bra, slippers, robe, toothbrush, toothpaste, hairbrush/comb, shampoo, hard candy and lip moisturizer for labor, other personal items, phone numbers of those to call, camera, clothes for mother to go home in, and clothes for baby to go home in (according to weather).

  b. When to call the OB provider

    1) Any signs and symptoms of illness, impending or premature labor

    2) When you have any question or concerns

  c. Family participation and visitation

    1) Know ahead of time the birth facility's visitation hours and family participation regulations.

    2) Plan ahead regarding the family's participation and visitation, during and after delivery.

CLASS III: CHILDBIRTH EDUCATION

1. Introduction

2. Labor review

   a. Contractions: Monitor for length, regularity, and duration. Monitor by feeling abdomen with fingertips, feeling for tightening and loosening.

      1) Timing contraction interval: Time from beginning of one contraction to the beginning of another contraction

      2) Timing contraction duration: Time from beginning of contraction to end of contraction

   b. True versus false: Labor is said to be true if it results in effacement and dilation.

   c. Premature: Before 37 weeks' gestation.

      1) Newborn complications related to preterm birth

         (a) Respiratory difficulty and increased chronic respiratory problems

         (b) More prone to illnesses and feeding problems

         (c) In general, all organs have not fully matured. All body systems are not functioning as well as those of a full-term, normal newborn, which subsequently causes the baby to have numerous problems, making the early months of lifedifficult.

      2) Prevention

         (a) Stop any smoking, drugs, alcohol

         (b) Eat balanced, nutritious meals; gain appropriate weight

         (c) Signs of premature labor: Any signs or symptoms of impending labor before 37 weeks

         (d) Intervention: Empty bladder; lie down on left side for at least 1 hour (increases oxygen to baby and uterus); drink at least 3 to 4 glasses of fluid while resting; feel abdomen and record pattern of contractions; if signs and symptoms do not cease, notify doctor/nurse-midwife with your name, due date, and signs and symptoms.

   d. Possible or actual signs and symptoms of impending labor

      1) Sudden burst of energy very soon before actual labor begins (nesting instinct)

      2) Lightening: the feeling that the baby has dropped lower in abdomen

      3) Discharge of pinkish mucus plug or unusual vaginal discharge

      4) Rupture of amniotic membrane (water breaks as a trickle or gush): Note color and any odor of amniotic fluid if not in hospital. If you even suspect your water has broken, go to the hospital.

5) Abdominal cramping, vaginal, thigh, or back pain or pressure

6) Regular contractions with or without pain over longer than 1 hour.

   (a) Contractions: Monitor for length, regularity, and duration. Monitor by feeling abdomen with fingertips, feeling for tightening and loosening.

   (b) Timing contraction interval: Time from beginning of one contraction to the beginning of another contraction

   (c) Timing contraction duration: Time from beginning of contraction to end of contraction

3. Relaxation and breathing practice

   a. Stages of labor: Breathing techniques (Detailed description is provided at the end of this chapter.)

      1) Stage I = dilation from 0 to 10 cm; three phases of Stage I

         (a) Early: Mild contractions, 0 to 5 cm dilation. Regular breathing to conserve energy with slow deep breath before/after each contraction. Coach should check for tense muscles and do gentle massage if mother desires (with flat hand—center to outer body). You can also incorporate any relaxation techniques that work for you throughout labor.

         (b) Active: Moderate contractions, 5 to 8 cm dilation. Pick focal point, concentrate on it throughout contraction, regular breathing increasing in speed, working into howt breathing as needed with the increase in pain.

         (c) Panting: 10 cm dilation. Just as it sounds; pant as if out of breath. OB provider may request this to help control delivery.

         Practice: Caution—do not push for real when practicing!

      2) Stage II: From 10 cm dilatation to birth of baby

         (a) Pushing: With contractions and provider direction, push, breathing deep breath in and out before contraction, deep breath in and hold, bear down with BM muscles for 10 seconds or as long as you can with the direction of the OB provider during the contraction, then deep cleansing breath after push to oxygenate you and the baby.

         Practice: Caution—do not push for real when practicing!

      3) Stage III: From birth of baby to delivery of placenta

4. Postpartum period (for the mother)

   a. Body Changes After Childbirth

      1) Reproductive Organs

         (a) "Shrinking" of uterus: Should be at the level of the navel and firm. If it is above the navel or feels spongy and soft, there is a much greater risk of increased bleeding. If the uterus is off to the side, your bladder is probably full. It should move down in the abdomen about one fingerbreadth/day, approaching nonpregnant size in 4 to 6 weeks.

(b) Lochia: Should be dark red for 2 to 3 days, pinkish brown for 3 to 10 days, creamy/yellowish for 1 to 2 weeks more. If clot is greater in size than a nickel, or unusual odor noted, or your bleeding gets heavier and darker, call your OB care provider.

(c) Cervix: closes slowly after birth

(d) Vagina: May be swollen and bruised. Do not use tampons or douches, because infection can occur.

(e) Perineum: May appear swollen and bruised. An episiotomy or laceration may be present with or without sutures. Ice can be used during the first 24 hours. Ask OB care provider about sitz baths before discharge.

(f) Recurrence of menses/ovulation: You will ovulate and can get pregnant before your first period occurs; recurrence of period varies person to person.

2) Abdomen

(a) Uterine ligaments and your abdominal wall have been stretched and need time to recover. Your abdomen may appear flabby for a time, but with exercise (and depending on your prepregnant condition), tone should return in 2 to 3 months. Consult with OB provider as to when you may begin to exercise.

(b) Stretch marks should lighten to silver/white appearance.

(c) If unusual tenderness or pain noted, notify OB provider immediately.

(d) Those delivering by cesarean may experience severe gas pain, which can be reduced by walking. Peppermint tea has been helpful to many women. OB provider can also prescribe or recommend remedy.

3) Lactation

(a) Regardless of whether you will be breastfeeding, your breasts have developed, and will begin to produce milk after birth of baby.

(b) If bottle feeding, breasts may get engorged and sore. To help reduce milk and promote "drying up," wear a supportive bra that fits well all the time, except for bathing. If the discomfort of swelling increases, use ice packs on chest and avoid hot showers hitting directly on breasts to prevent increased swelling.

(c) Breastfeeding information (See Parent Teaching Information in this manual)

(d) Provides increased, special immunities to help protect the baby from infection that only mother can provide when the baby is more vulnerable.

(e) Always consult your clinician or pharmacist before taking any type of medication in any form if you are breastfeeding. It may affect the baby.

4) Gastrointestinal

   (a) Mother is usually very hungry and thirsty after labor and should be able to eat (unless she has delivered by cesarean, in which oral food will be withheld until bowel sounds return).

   (b) First bowel movement may be delayed. Many mothers will fear tearing their stitches and wait to have bowel movement, but this will increase chance of constipation and discomfort; stool softeners may also help.

   (c) Flatus is common, especially after cesarean. Flatus results especially after cesarean because of manipulation of intestines during surgery, resulting in temporary decreased motility. Early ambulation and "anti-gas" medication will help relieve this.

5) Urinary Tract

   (a) May have decreased sensation of need to void, and overfilling of bladder is possible. Be sure to attempt to void every few hours; notify OB care provider if unable to void, there is burning with urination, blood in the urine, or if urine is cloudy or foul smelling.

   (b) May experience slight incontinence when active. This is common because of decreased tone of voiding muscles. Kegel exercises will help strengthen these muscles and decrease leaking.

6) Temperature

   (a) A temperature up to 100.4 F is normal within the first 24 hours. If fever is present after that, notify clinician.

7) Weight Loss

   (a) Initial loss can be 10 to 12 lbs after birth.

   (b) Five pounds may be lost soon after birth because of increased urination and excretion of extra fluid.

   (c) After 5 to 6 weeks, you should be near prepregnant weight if you gained 25 to 30 lbs and maintain an appropriate diet.

8) Postpartum chill

   (a) Women sometimes experience a "shaking chill" shortly after delivery. This is normal and fine, as long as it is not accompanied by continued fever (a warm beverage and blankets often help).

9) Postpartum sweating

   (a) Increased sweating after birth occurs to eliminate extra water and waste products from the body (and often occurs at night).

10) Afterpains

(a) Caused by intermittent uterine contraction

(b) Increased in women who have had more than one child

(c) May cause little to severe discomfort 2 to 3 days after birth

(d) If Pitocin given after birth to help with uterine firmness, this will increase discomfort.

(e) Breastfeeding often stimulates afterpains.

(f) Rocking in a chair, or propping a pillow under abdomen while lying on your side may assist with discomfort.

11) Breasts

(a) Often enlarged and sore, often leak breast milk, but if a reddened area noted, notify clinician.

(b) If breastfeeding, watch breasts for cracking and open sores; increased chance of infection

(c) Interventions for common breast discomforts in Chapter 8, Postpartum Instructions

12) Skin

(a) If tearing or episiotomy occurred, sutures may be present. Be alert for any bleeding from suture site (do not confuse with lochia), any unusual drainage, odor, separation of skin at injured site, or pressure in that area. If so, notify clinician.

13) Extremities

(a) If swelling of legs or ankles occurred during pregnancy, it should resolve. If new swelling, tenderness, or redness noted in legs (especially if just one), let clinician know.

14) Postpartum guidelines for mothers (See Parent Teaching Information)

b. Psychological changes after childbirth

1) Adjustment to all the new changes, new roles the family will play; this may cause many different emotions.

2) Postpartum blues: Occurs in some women in different degrees, as a temporary depression lasting usually 1 to 2 weeks after birth, and may be experienced in many different ways (being cranky, crying at commercials). Do not be afraid to talk out your feelings with someone, family, friend, or clinician. It often helps.

3) Cultural influences: Different cultures have different rituals they follow after mother has the baby.

4) Attachment: The process of interaction and bonding between mother and baby

c. Health supervision

1) Woman's 6-week postpartum checkup

(a) Make sure you attend to ensure your health. Moms often put off their own health care.

(b) If you have any signs of illness, especially a temperature greater than 100.0 F, chills, abdominal pain, increased bleeding, large clots, dizziness, continued headaches, continued swelling in legs, do not wait for checkup. Call clinician immediately.

(c) Discuss the type of contraception you will use with your clinician. You will be informed of options, risks, and appropriate time to begin.

(d) Remember that you will ovulate, and therefore will be able to get pregnant before you see your next period. Breastfeeding will NOT prevent pregnancy.

(e) If you used a diaphragm, you must be reevaluated for one because your vagina is no longer the same size, and the diaphragm may not be effective.

(f) Your clinician will recommend when it is safe to resume intercourse. Condoms are recommended to prevent infection.

5. Postpartum period (for the infant)
   a. Physical care
      1) Health
         (a) Resting: The baby will get much stimulation from new relatives and friends and will need plenty of rest. You can tell the baby needs a break from stimulation when she looks away from you when you attempt to play, is irritable, etc.
      2) Breathing
         (a) The baby should normally breathe 30 to 60 times per minute. This breathing will have an irregular pattern (slow then fast), so count respirations for a full minute to assess if the breathing is out of range.
         (b) Babies breathe much of the time through their noses, so keep the nares as uncongested as possible with bulb syringe.
         (c) Babies may have short periods when they are breathing very slowly. If this pause lasts longer than 15 seconds, let clinician know.
         (d) Respiratory distress (baby is not getting enough oxygen) has many symptoms: blueness around the mouth, faster breathing, grunting sound to breathing, nostrils flaring, baby agitated or less responsive. Call 911 immediately.
         (e) A cardiopulmonary resuscitation (CPR) class (often occur frequently in many locations) will teach what to do if baby stops breathing, chokes, or heart stops beating. CPR classes are offered frequently in many locations.
      3) Temperature
         (a) Monitor temperature at home (normal, 97 to 99 F) to get to know baby's normal temperature.

    (b) Dress baby appropriately for weather (same number of layers or one more layer of clothing than you are wearing). Overdressing can cause an increased body temperature.

    (c) Keep baby well covered during bathing to prevent excessive heat loss.

4) Hydration–Nutrition

    (a) Provide the recommended formula (unless breastfeeding) and amount (often this is based on infant demand).

    (b) If breastfeeding, be sure to have infant on each breast for an equal amount of time, to ensure breast stimulation by infant is adequate for milk production.

    (c) Baby will lose some weight the first week. Babies are born with extra fluid that they use while waiting for milk supply, which appears usually around the third day. This is nature's protection for them.

    (d) Monitor for symptoms of dehydration, especially if infant is experiencing decreased intake, vomiting, or diarrhea (dry mouth, decreased urination, stronger-smelling and darker urine, increased temperature) and notify clinician immediately.

5) Safety

    (a) Always use a carseat. Make sure it fits in your car correctly and fits the size of the baby.

    (b) Frequent hand washing by all persons near baby is very helpful in preventing infection. Those who are sick should limit contact with the baby. Appropriate cleaning of all baby equipment is important.

    (c) Signs of general illness in baby include vomiting, diarrhea, elevated temperature, congestion, coughing, dehydration, and continued irritability.

    (d) Appropriate cord care is important. Use alcohol to clean around the cord until it comes off, monitor for any signs of redness, swelling, drainage, or foul odor at cord site. This could be an infection.

6) Health supervision

    (a) The baby should be taken to all scheduled medical appointments to ensure normal health, growth, and development. These appointments should include the regular immunizations, which prevent serious illness.

    (b) Postpartum newborn record

b. Psychological care

1) This is the time for bonding and attachment between parents and baby. As you are meeting the needs of the infant (food, comfort, safety, affection), the emotional bond of trust is strengthened between you, and adversely, if the basic needs of infant are often not met, this bond is hindered.

2) From the time the infant is born, it begins to learn. Everything it feels, smells, sees, and hears is integrated into its being, be it good or bad. Even the most basic of activities is a learning experience and promotes development of the infant. The more stimulation he or she receives, the more she or he learns.

Breathing Techniques

1. Early labor (0 to 5 cm)
   a. Deep, relaxing breaths, in through the nose, out through the mouth. Think about blowing away the contraction.

2. Active labor (5 to 8 cm) and transitional labor (8 to 10 cm)
   a. Howt: Short, faster, rhythmic breathing. Use high chest muscles to inhale and exhale. Inhale on "How," begin exhale on "w," and finish exhaling on "t." Accentuate "t" on exhale to avoid buildup of carbon dioxide and risk of fainting. Start and finish with a deep, relaxing breath.
   b. Howt breathing requires some practice. It also requires concentration to maintain in labor during a contraction, reducing the woman's ability to concentrate on fear or pain. The brain's response to fear and pain can cause a reduction in blood flow to the uterus (physiologic fight-or-flight reaction).

3. Panting (10 cm)
   a. Panting breaths are best described as being like an overheated canine. These are used to help control the actual delivery.

4. Pushing (10 cm): DO NOT TRULY PUSH DURING PRACTICE! ONLY PUSH WHEN OB PROVIDER INSTRUCTS YOU TO DO SO!
   a. Take a deep, relaxing breath in and out at first feeling of contraction beginning. Inhale deeply and hold, while bringing chin down to chest.
   b. Push while holding your breath, using the same muscles as those you use to have a bowel movement. (Use of the abdominal muscles is ineffective.)
   c. Attempt to hold breath while pushing to the count of 10. Release breath and quickly repeat entire process. Attempt to get three pushes with each contraction.

Fetal Behavior and Movement

The fetus is active and responsive. Fetal mobility occurs early, but the mother's perception of fetal movement (quickening) does not occur until 16 to 20 weeks in first-time mothers, and 14 to 16 weeks in later pregnancies. Fetal behavior is influenced by its state of sleep or alertness. The actual number of daily movements is variable between fetuses; thus it is important for the mother to establish what is normal for her baby before any problems arise. Box 7-1 provides a guideline to the stages of fetal movement. Figure 7-1 is a Sample Fetal Movement Record a woman might use to track her fetus' movements.

![] RECOMMENDED TEXT

Reeder S.J., Martin L.L. & Koniak-Griffin, D. (1997). *Maternity Nursing: Family, Newborn, and Women's Health*, 18th ed. Philadelphia: Lippincott-Raven Publishers.

![] RECOMMENDED RESOURCES FOR EDUCATIONAL TOOLS

Childbirth Graphics
P.O. Box 21207
Waco, TX 76702-1207

Miracle of Life, Nova series, produced for the Corporation for Public Broadcasting by Films for the Humanities and Sciences, Monmouth Junction, NJ, 1-800-257-5126.

CHAPTER 8

Client–Family Teaching Handouts

The material found in this section of the manual is meant to be copied and distributed to clients and their families to assist in teaching. These are just a few of the teaching materials one can access with a little research. Excellent materials can be found through The Division of Maternal Child Health, Health and Human Services, 4350 East West Highway, Rockville, MD 20857. In addition, further resources should be available through your state and local health departments. Visual and written aids assist the nurse in the educational process by stimulating multiple senses in the student and thus increasing memory stimulation.

These items are exactly what they claim to be—tools. They are meant to assist the nurse in the educational process. They are not a substitute for the nurse–client relationship that develops as a result of practicing the art of nursing empathy. The nurse should always take the time to review these handouts with clients. Do not assume that your client can read or has developed an adequate trusting relationship to value your information.

Nurses in home care work in the domain of the client, not the office or hospital. The client maintains more control of "the helping relationship" in home care because the nurse works on the client's "turf." The nurse's ability to communicate and develop the helping relationship is crucial to successful practice of home health nursing.

Preterm Labor

What is preterm labor and what does it mean to your baby? Now that your OB care provider has diagnosed preterm labor, you probably have many questions. This information is provided to help you understand the diagnosis of preterm labor as well as to help you identify more questions that you might want to ask your OB care provider or nurse. The information here will also attempt to help you understand and deal with the treatment plan you might need to follow.

What Does Preterm Mean?

Pregnancy is calculated to be 40 weeks from the first day of your last period. Any delivery beyond the 37th week is considered term. Any delivery that occurs during the period of 20 to 36 weeks is considered preterm. Preterm birth is one of the most important problems affecting newborns today. Some of the complications include respiratory difficulties, feeding problems, infections, and problems with temperature regulation. This is why it is so important to provide this information to you, so that you can have the tools to help identify, treat, and prevent preterm labor and birth.

Am I at Risk?

The cause of preterm labor and birth is not exactly understood, but certain situations have been identified as increasing your risk for preterm labor. The following have been associated with an increased risk of preterm labor:

1. Previous preterm labor or delivery
2. Abnormally shaped uterus, DES daughters, uterine surgery
3. Two or more second trimester abortions or miscarriages
4. Incompetent cervix, cone biopsy, large fibroids
5. Current pregnancy with twins, triplets, etc.
6. Feeling that something is wrong, even without any specific symptoms or cause

How Can I Check for Contractions?

Lie down and place your fingers on your uterus. If your uterus is tightening and softening you will be able to tell how often it is happening. Time the contractions by noting the time between the start of one tightening and the start of the next tightening. Because at times uterine contractions (especially in preterm labor) occur without any other warning signs, it is important that you feel your abdomen for contractions (or use home monitoring if that is part of your treatment) at least twice a day for half-hour periods. It is very helpful to do this at the same time each day if possible.

How Will I Be Treated If I Have Preterm Labor?

Sometimes preterm labor may be treated with rest and modification of your activities. You might need to increase your rest time. Rest on your side at least twice a day in the morning and afternoon. You might need to modify or stop work or school activities. You will need to discuss with your OB care provider or nurse how long your rest period needs to be. Many times bed rest at home is recommended. That can be more difficult than you could imagine. You will need to adjust many aspects of your life. The temporary reorganization of your activities might need to include stopping work, managing your household from bed, reorganizing your house, and assisting with the care of your children.

An excellent book available to you that contains lots of practical ideas and answers to many questions is *Pregnancy Bed Rest*—a guide for the pregnant woman and her family written by Susan H. Johnson and Deborah A. Kraut. This book is available at your local bookstore.

Will I Have to Be Admitted to the Hospital?

Sometimes you might need to be hospitalized and treated with medications for your preterm labor. Medications that will be used are called tocolytics (Brethine (terbutaline), Yutopar (ritodrine), or magnesium sulfate). These medications stop labor by relaxing the muscles of the uterus. Like many medications, they will affect your body with additional side effects:

1. You may experience a faster heartbeat, tremors, nausea, vomiting, headache, and flushing of the skin.
2. You might experience other symptoms, such as nervousness, jitteriness, restlessness, anxiety, tiredness, listlessness, stomach discomforts, difficulty in breathing, drowsiness, and weakness, but these are less common.

(continued)

It is very important that you discuss the medications with your OB care provider or nurse so that you know exactly what you are taking, how often you should take your medication, and what to expect with the particular medication you are taking. It is possible to receive tocolytic medication via a small pump that delivers the medication under your skin. The use of this pump allows for very small amounts of medication to be delivered more frequently.

The feelings that you might experience can range anywhere from fear, tremendous guilt, to anger and frustration. Many women report feeling numb and helpless as the diagnosis is first presented to them. Many ask, "Why me? What have I done to deserve this?" Your expectations and hopes for your unborn child can often change into incredible fear for the health of your baby. You will probably always feel a sense of threat to the pregnancy and often wonder if you will be a mother of a healthy baby. You might at times also feel inadequate because you might not be able to maintain a safe environment for your baby. All of these feelings are very normal and are very common in women experiencing preterm labor or high risk pregnancy.

The feelings of the loss of the "perfect pregnancy" and the guilt from believing that you somehow have caused preterm labor are experienced by many women. It is important that you understand that these feelings are very normal in your situation and that you are not the only person who has ever felt like this. It might be helpful for you to discuss your feelings with your OB care provider or nurse. The father of the new baby may experience the same fears and concerns for you and the baby. He is often asked to be the main source of emotional support for you and your family. Many fathers feel jealous and guilty at the same time. The feelings of jealousy toward the baby and your preoccupation with the pregnancy are many times accompanied by feelings of guilt over these feelings. Fathers many times will feel protective of their wives and at the same time anxious about whether they will be able to provide the care that their partner and baby might need.

The effect of your hospitalization on your family can be tremendous. Family members might feel left out in the "high tech" care environment of the hospital. It is important that you enlist their care and support, as much as they are able to provide for you. It is also very important that you attempt to spend as much time as possible with your children to help them maintain their feeling of importance to the family. Discussion of all of your feelings between you and your partner as well as with the family is very important to the protection of your family unit.

Kegel Exercises

The primary muscle involved is the pubococcygeus (P-C) muscle. When exercised, the P-C muscle:

1. Strengthens urinary sphincter control
2. Increases your muscle tone in the vagina
3. Increases your ability to constrict the vagina voluntarily. This increases female vaginal perception and response during penile–vaginal intercourse
4. Contributes to elimination of pain during sexual intercourse
5. Aids in birth of baby by increasing your ability to relax the pelvic floor.
6. Aids in postpartum recovery of tone of pelvic floor muscles

To identify the P-C muscle, sit on the toilet with your legs spread as far apart as possible. Start and stop the flow of urine. The P-C muscle is the only one that can accomplish this while in this position.

Practice the Kegel exercise 5 times a day (15 contractions each time) or 10 contractions whenever you open the refrigerator. Soon Kegels will become second nature to you. Contract the P-C muscle, hold for 3 seconds, relax, and repeat the process.

Because the P-C is a muscle like other muscles, with too much strenuous exercise it can become sore. If this happens, either stop doing the exercise for 1 or 2 days until the temporary soreness disappears and then resume, or reduce substantially the amount of exercise per day, and gradually increase it to the recommended number.

Once you learn where the muscles are, the Kegel exercise can be done during daily activities that do not involve a great deal of moving around (eg, driving an automobile, sitting, doing dishes, watching TV, waiting in a checkout line, lying in bed).

Postpartum Instructions for Mothers

The following information is to be used as a guideline for instructing mothers and families to care for themselves and their newborns. The mother should be instructed as follows (unless otherwise instructed by their primary care provider):

A. Rest
1. Get plenty of rest for a couple of weeks after birth.
2. Focus on care for self and baby; do not expect much of yourself.
3. Obtain help for general household duties (cleaning, cooking, laundry, shopping, and caring for older children).
4. Try to rest when the baby is sleeping.
5. Limit visitors to relatives and close friends. Make sure everyone washes hands before touching the baby to prevent the spread of infection.
6. Remember, fatigue decreases your milk supply and your ability to cope with new and added responsibilities.

B. Activity
1. Limit stair climbing for the first week.
2. Resume your normal activity and exercise very gradually over 6 weeks.
3. You may go out to dinner or for a ride but do not drive for 1 to 2 weeks unless otherwise instructed by physician. If you delivered your baby by cesarean section, verify with your OB care provider about when driving is permitted.

C. Diet
1. Drink 8 to 10 glasses of water per day.
2. Eat plenty of proteins, fruits, and vegetables, and drink plenty of milk.
3. A small bowl of bran daily will prevent constipation.
4. Ask your primary care provider if you should continue taking prenatal vitamins daily.
5. An adequate diet as shown above is important especially if you are breastfeeding. It takes about 800 calories a day to produce the milk the baby needs.
6. Remember, if you do not eat, you will become fatigued, and milk volume will decrease.

D. Vaginal Discharge
1. At first the discharge is red, like a heavy period, for about 1 to 3 days.
2. By the 3rd day, the discharge should have thinned and lightened in color.
3. By the 10th day, the discharge is often a pale pink, watery fluid, but still heavy enough to wear a light pad.
4. If after the 3rd day bleeding becomes bright red and heavy again, it is often a sign that you have done too much and you should slow down and rest.

E. Intercourse
1. For most women, intercourse may be resumed when the vaginal area feels comfortable and your episiotomy has healed. You should check any doubts you have with your physician.
2. Gentleness and added lubrication may be needed for comfort when you first resume sexual activity.
3. Breastfeeding mothers may ovulate before their first menstrual period; therefore, it is possible to get pregnant even before menstruation has resumed.
4. Foam and condoms will provide contraception if sexual activity is resumed before 6 weeks postpartum.
5. Birth control should be discussed at the 6-week postpartum visit.

F. Baths and Showers
1. You may shower as necessary but DO NOT take a tub bath for at least 3 days unless otherwise instructed by OB care provider. DO NOT use bubble bath or oils in bath water.
2. Warm showers may help to relieve the discomfort of breast engorgement.
3. DO NOT USE DOUCHES! They can cause trauma and possible infection.

G. Stiches and Hemorrhoids
1. Warm tub baths or sitz bath are recommended several times a day.
2. For discomfort of hemorrhoids, Nupercainol cream, Dermoplast, or Tucks pads may be helpful. Consult your OB care provider.
3. Do not become alarmed if a week or two postpartum, loose stitches are found on a pad or in the toilet.
4. Stitches are normally absorbed or loosen when they are no longer needed.

(continued)

H. Postpartum Blues
   1. You may experience "postpartum blues" during the first 10 days postpartum. The most common symptom is unexpected and unexplainable crying. You also may feel irritable.
   2. Postpartum blues usually go away in about 72 hours, but may continue for as long as 10 days.
   3. You may be experiencing postpartum depression if the postpartum blues symptoms persist or increase in severity after 10 days.
   4. Postpartum depression is experienced by 10% of all women and may occur anywhere within the time 6 months after delivery.
   5. Signs and symptoms of postpartum depression may include any or all of the following:
      a. Sleep disturbance
      b. Loss of appetite
      c. Fear and anxiety
      d. Hopelessness
      e. Hostility or self-blame
      f. Difficulty concentrating or making decisions
   6. You should seek professional help if signs and symptoms of postpartum depression are experienced.

I. Postpartum Problems:

CALL YOUR HEALTH CARE PROVIDER IF ANY OF THE FOLLOWING PROBLEMS OCCUR:

   1. A flulike feeling, fever, or chills
   2. Foul-smelling discharge or unusual abdominal tenderness
   3. Redness or tenderness of breasts
   4. Extreme tenderness of episiotomy area
   5. Tenderness of pubic bone, accompanied by frequency, urgency, and burning with urination.

These symptoms may indicate an infection of some type, which requires immediate professional attention and treatment.

Newborn Instructions

Relax with your infant. He/she will adjust to you. If you are tense, baby will feel tense; if you are relaxed, it will help relax your baby.

A. Bathing
   1. Sponge bathe with mild soap (low alkaline) such as Dove or Castille, until the umbilical cord has fallen off and is completely healed.
   2. Do not use oil or powder on baby's head or skin.
   3. When the navel is healed, baby may have a tub bath.
   4. Bathe baby before feeding.

B. Cord Care
   1. The umbilical cord usually falls off within 7 to 10 days.
   2. Use alcohol and cotton to cleanse and bathe the area around the base of the cord at every diaper change.
   3. There may be one or two drops of blood when the cord separates.
   4. Keep the diaper folded beneath the naval to facilitate drying.
   5. Call the pediatric care provider if the cord has a foul odor or if the skin of the abdominal area and the umbilical cord becomes red.

C. Diaper Rash
   1. Change baby's diaper as soon as possible when soiled.
   2. Avoid using plastic pants when possible or change baby frequently. Air buttocks when changing.
   3. Cloth diapers should be washed with mild soap and rinsed well after each laundering.
   4. Apply a diaper rash ointment, such as Balmex or Desitin, to the diaper area, especially to the creases, at each diaper change (Vaseline can be used all the time on diaper area).

D. Circumcision
   1. Apply Vaseline liberally at every diaper change until the area is no longer red or swollen.
   2. Signs and symptoms of infection include increasing instead of decreasing amount of redness and swelling, and yellowish/greenish pus. The healing penis will present smegma, a whitish material adhering to the circumcised area. This does not wipe off as pus does.

E. Nails
   1. Use an emery board to file the nails. They are too soft to cut with scissors for the first couple of weeks.
   2. Never cut with cuticle scissors.

F. Clothing
   1. Keep the baby warm but do not overheat.
   2. Use simple, easily washed clothes.
   3. On hot days,a diaper and tee-shirt may be enough.
   4. The baby should wear the same number or one more layer of clothing than his/her mother.
   5. If it is cool and breezy, the baby's head should be covered.

G. Feeding
   1. If breastfeeding, refer to instructions and information on breastfeeding.
   2. Hold baby at every feeding—do not prop the bottle.
   3. Feed baby whenever he/she is hungry (usually every 3 to 5 hours, more if breastfed).
   4. Do not wake baby at night to eat.
   5. Burp the baby after every 1/2 to 1 oz. for the first week and then every 1 to 2 oz.
   6. Place baby on his/her back or side (roll blanket and place behind back for support).
   7. Do not start any new foods (cereal, juice, or fruit) until your pediatric provider gives permission.
   8. If bottlefeeding, use formula as ordered by pediatric provider. Powdered form may be more economical. The client should always follow instructions on the can for mixing and preparing the powdered formula.
   9. May have 1 to 2 oz. of boiled, cooled water in between feedings if fussy, but newborns do not need water and should not receive more than 2 oz., because too much water can cause hyponatremia.

H. Bowel Movements
   1. Breastfed baby's bowel movements are normally loose and unformed.
   2. Breastfed baby may have several small bowel movements each day or go for several days without having a bowel movement at all.
   3. A totally breastfed baby is never constipated and seldom has diarrhea (watery bowel movements).

(continued)

I. Fussy Periods
   1. May go through fussy periods during the day or evening.
   2. May happen because mother's milk supply is low at the end of the day.
   3. May need to nurse more frequently.
   4. Use calming tactics such as rocking, walking, strollers, swings, etc.
   5. Lay baby down to see if he/she will sleep.

J. Rest
   1. Babies show their individual personalities immediately. No baby does exactly what the instructions say they should. Some babies will sleep and eat more than others. On average, though, bottlefed babies tend to eat every 3 to 4 hours. Breastfed babies eat a little more frequently. Newborns usually sleep in between their feedings, increasing their awake time just a little each day. The most important thing for all new families is to relax and get to know their new little individual in the family and his/her own needs.

K. Reducing the Risk of Sudden Infant Death Syndrome
   1. Babies should be placed down to sleep on their backs or on their sides with the lower arm forward to stop them from rolling over. For more information, call Back to Sleep Campaign at 1-800-505-CRIB, or you can write to Back to Sleep, P.O. Box 29111, Washington, DC 20040.

Breastfeeding

A. Positioning for Breastfeeding
1. Assume a comfortable position (sitting, lying, football hold). Positions should be rotated to avoid stress or sore nipples.
2. Bring baby to nipple. You may want to use pillows because this will avoid stress of the baby pulling on your nipples.
3. Expose breast, support the baby's head in the crook of the arm, with the other hand supporting the nipple in a scissors-like or thumb and forefinger hold.
4. Compress breast if it is large, with finger at baby's nose, to prevent obstruction of baby's breathing.
5. Timing
   a. 5 minutes first day, per breast
   b. 7 to 8 minutes second day, per breast
   c. 10 minutes third day, per breast. Build up to 20 minutes per breast.
   d. If baby falls asleep after 10 minutes when milk comes in, cut back to 5 minutes per breast.
   e. If baby is still hungry, may go back to first breast for another 5 minutes.
   f. Nurse both breasts at each feeding. Start with breast ended with at the last feeding.
   g. At end of feeding, break suction by placing finger in corner of baby's mouth.
   h. Air-dry nipples after each feeding and apply Eucerin cream around areola (brown area) but not on the tip of the nipple. This will help keep nipples from becoming tender.

B. Breast Massage and Hand Expression
1. Must be used to bring milk down to the baby, to relieve fullness, and before pumping or hand expressing to decrease the time spent on collection.
2. To massage: Place one hand under breast, with other hand stroke down toward the nipple, starting from the shoulder down, under breast, and then up. Do this for 1 minute on each breast.
3. To hand express, put thumb and forefinger on areola about 1 inch from nipple. Press back toward the chest wall and squeeze together to compress milk sinus.

C. Milk Collection and Storage
1. This may be done when mothers work or are not going to be home for feedings and want the baby to drink from a bottle.
2. Collect by hand expression, breast pump, or with milk cups.
3. Collect in a clean container; label container with date milk was expressed.
4. Glass, plastic bottles, or double-bagged nursers may be used.
5. Chill, then freeze. Pour chilled milk on top of frozen.
6. May store in refrigerator 24 to 48 hours only.
7. Milk can be kept in back of freezer for several months.
8. To defrost, run under cold, then warm water, then shake.
9. Discard defrosted milk that the baby does not use.
10. Milk to be transported should be placed in an insulated bag, frozen, or packed with ice.
11. Storage
    a. Milk may be kept at room temperature.
       1) Colostrum: 12 to 24 hours
       2) Mature milk: 6 to 10 hours
    b. Hospitalized infants: Milk should be refrigerated within 1 hour of expressing.
    c. Milk may be refrigerated:
       1) Mature milk up to 5 days
       2) Hospitalized infants up to 48 hours
    d. Milk may be frozen for
       1) 2 weeks in a freezer compartment located inside a refrigerator
       2) 6 months in a separate door refrigerator/freezer (frost free) (3 months for hospitalized infants)
       3) 6 months to 1 year in deep freezer, 0 F or below
    e. Warming milk
       1) Thaw or heat by placing container in warm water; human milk heats to a comfortable feeding temperature in about 10 minutes.
       2) Shake before testing temperature.

(continued)

D. Expressing Breastmilk
   1. Breastmilk may be expressed and collected for later use by using hand expression, a hand-operated breast pump, or a semiautomatic battery-operated or electric breast pump.
   2. A sterile container such as sterile plastic "bottle bags" (Playtex or Gerber liners) or a sterilized plastic or glass bottle should be used to collect the milk.
   3. Before collecting milk, wash hands with soap and water, then dry hands thoroughly.
   4. Massage each breast in the following way:
      a. If large-breasted, support the breast with one hand. Beginning at the chest wall, use the other flattened hand to exert gentle pressure on the breast toward the nipple, working around the breast. Work in areas of greatest milk duct development: under the breast and along the side under the arm. Use palms of hands, not fingers, for firm pressure. (Alaska Department of Health, Maternal Child Public Health Manual, Vol. 2, Maternal Health, 1995.)
   5. Stimulate the "let-down reflex" or "milk ejection reflex" by gently rolling and tugging the nipples between thumb and forefinger.
   6. Dripping of milk from the nipples is one sign that the let-down or milk ejection reflex is working. When you feel that the let-down reflex has begun to work, you can begin expressing breastmilk through whichever method you choose.
   7. Collecting milk may take about 20 minutes. Alternate the breast from which you are expressing milk about four times in this fashion: when milk flow slows down on one breast, go to the other breast.
   8. A breast pump collection kit should be washed daily in soap and water, rinsed between uses. A dishwasher (which leaves no soap residue) provides an excellent method for cleaning the kit (when collecting milk for a hospitalized infant, the collection kit must be sterilized daily).

E. Breastfeeding Problems and Solutions
   1. Nipple Soreness
      a. Problem: Nipples may become red and cracked or bleeding. Nipples may be sore until they become accustomed to the baby's sucking. Soreness may also be due to poor positioning, removing baby from breast improperly, not allowing the nipples to dry, irritants such as soap, shampoo, rough clothing, plastic liners in bras, or harsh laundry detergents.
      b. Solutions
         1) Rotate position of baby when feeding
         2) Short frequent feedings
         3) Make sure baby has large portion of nipple in mouth, not just the tip
         4) Make sure baby's mouth is close to the nipple to avoid pulling on the nipple
         5) Air-dry nipples and use Eucerin cream as necessary
         6) Nurse on least sore side first
         7) Always break suction before removing baby
         8) Apply saline soaks, ice to nipples before feeding, nipple shields, or vitamin E oil if nipples become cracked or bleeds
   2. Fullness or engorgement
      a. Problem: Breasts become full on 2nd or 3rd day postpartum when milk comes in. Engorgement is when milk becomes backed up and the breast and nipples become hard and shiny.
      b. Solutions
         1) Short, frequent feedings. Do not miss feedings. Nurse on both sides each feeding.
         2) Warm showers, compresses, massages, and expression relieve fullness.
         3) Make sure bra is not cutting or binding in any place.
         4) May occasionally express or pump after feeding to relieve fullness.
   3. Plugged duct
      a. Problem: Lump or tenderness in one spot.
      b. Solution
         1) Nurse on affected breast first.
         2) Direct baby's chin toward lump when nursing.
         3) Avoid tight bras, underwire bras, and bunching clothing.
         4) Use massage and heat while nursing to encourage lump drainage.
   4. Breast infection
      a. Problem: Symptoms include flulike feeling, redness, tenderness, and fever. This may be aggravated by not emptying the breast completely, abrupt weaning, or fatigue.

(continued)

  b. Solutions
    1) Heat—warm, moist compresses
    2) Rest
    3) Empty breast—when nursing, direct baby's chin toward sore spot or lump
    4) If temperature increases to 100 F, call physician
5. Growth spurts
  a. Growth spurts are short periods of rapid cellular growth for the newborn and usually come within the first 10 days, 3 weeks, 3 months, and 6 months.
  b. Baby may want to nurse more often as metabolism increases.
  c. Nurse baby on demand to build up milk supply.
  d. Do not give supplemental formula feeding, because this will interfere with necessary milk production. The frequent nursing is necessary to stimulate the production of a greater supply of breast milk to meet the increased metabolic needs of the growing infant.

Bibliography

Alaska Department of Health and Social Services: *Alaska Maternal and Child Health Manual for Public Health Nursing.* Alaska Department of Health and Social Services, Division of Public Health, Section of Nursing, Anchorage, Alaska; June 1994.

American Diabetes Association: *Medical Management of Pregnancy Complicated by Diabetes.* American Diabetes Association, Alexandria, Virginia; 1993.

Arkin, Elaine Bratic, and Judith E. Funkhouser: *Communicating About Alcohol and Other Drugs: Strategies for Reaching Populations at Risk.* U.S. Department of Public Health and Human Services, Rockville, Maryland; 1990.

Association of Maternal and Child Health Programs: *Caring for Mothers and Children. A Report of a Survey of FY 1987 State MCH Program Activities.* Association of Maternal and Child Health Programs, Washington, D.C.; March 1989.

Association of Maternal and Child Health Programs: *Toward the Future of Title V! A Report on Site Visits to Ten State Programs.* Association of Maternal and Child Health Programs, Washington, D.C.; November 1991.

Association of Maternal and Child Health Programs: *Meeting Needs, Building Capacities. State Perspectives on Graduate Training and Continuing Education Needs of Title V Programs.* Association of Maternal and Child Health Programs, Washington, D.C.; October 1992.

Association of Women's Health, Obstetric, and Neonatal Nurses: *Practice Resource: Preparation for Technology-Dependent Infants.* Association of Women's Health, Obstetric, and Neonatal Nurses; McLean, Virginia, January 1993.

Bass, Alison: Few support services are available once ill children go home. *Boston Sunday Globe*, November 27, 1988.

Betz, Cecily Lynn, et al.: Altered digestive function. *Family Centered Nursing Care of Infants*, 35:1478–1480; 1994.

Block, Carol, et al.: *Home Care for High-Risk Infants, The First Year. Caring*, pp. 11–17. National Association for Home Care, Washington, D.C.; May 1989.

Boland, Mary G., and Lynn Czarniecki: Starting life with HIV, *RN*, pp. 54–58; January 1991.

Boyer, D.: Prediction of postpartum depression. *NAACOG Clinical Issues in Perinatal and Women's Health Nursing*, 1(3):267–278; 1990.

Bradley, Robert, and Bettye Caldwell: Using the HOME inventory to assess the family environment. *Pediatric Nursing*, 14(2)97-102; March–April 1988.

Briggs, Nancy: Hospitals & home care: Inseparable in the '80's. *Pediatric Nursing*, 12(5):384–385; September–October 1986.

Briggs, Nancy, Connie Lierman, Julie Hazelton, Richard Wolff, Kinny Pasquera, and Elizabeth Wilson: Multidisciplinary treatment of feeding disorders in the home. *Pediatric Nursing*, 13(4):266–271; July–August 1987.

Britton, John R., and Helen Britton: Efficacy of early newborn discharge in a middle-class population. *MDC*, 138:1041–1045; November 1984.

Britton, John R., Helen Britton, and Susan Beebe: Early discharge of the term newborn: A continued dilemma. *Pediatrics*, 94(3):291–295; September 1994.

Brown, Sarah S., ed.: *Prenatal Care. Reaching Mothers. Reaching Infants.* National Academy Press, Washington, D.C.; 1988.

Casey, Robert P.: *Investing in Our Children and Families, 1993–94 Budget Initiatives.* Executive Office, Harrisburg, Pennsylvania 1993.

Casey, Robert P.: *Managed Competition: A Health Care System for Pennsylvania.* Report of the Pennsylvania Economic Development Partnership Health Care Committee to The Pennsylvania Economic Development Partnership. Executive Office, Harrisburg, Pennsylvania; November 1992.

Child Health Foundation: Diarrhea kills over 300 U.S. children annually. *NEWS, Child Health Foundation Newsletter*, Columbia, Maryland; June 2, 1996.

Children's Hospital of Los Angeles: *Informational Guidelines for Parents.* Children's Hospital of Los Angeles, Nutrition Support Program, Los Angeles; 1990.

Children's Hospital of Philadelphia: *Informational Guidelines for Parents.* Children's Hospital of Philadelphia, Nutrition Support Program, Philadelphia; 1991.

Commonwealth of Pennsylvania, Department of Health: *Maternal and Child Health Services.* Draft Block Grant Application, Federal Fiscal Year 1993. Pennsylvania Department of Health, Harrisburg, Pennsylvania 1993.

Commonwealth of Pennsylvania, Department of Health: *Guide to Health Data for Pennsylvania.* State Health Data Center, Harrisburg, Pennsylvania; June 1996.

Commonwealth of Pennsylvania, Department of Public Welfare: *Pennsylvania Medical Assistance Program Eligibility Verification System Manual.* Publication 261. Pennsylvania Department of Public Welfare, Harrisburg, Pennsylvania; April 1993.

Commonwealth of Pennsylvania, Department of Public Welfare: Statistics provided by outpatient staff. Pennsylvania Department of Public Welfare, Harrisburg, Pennsylvania; May 13, 1993.

Commonwealth of Pennsylvania, Department of Public Welfare: *Overview, The Family Care Network.* Pennsylvania Department of Public Welfare, Harrisburg, Pennsylvania; 1994.

Cook, Paddy, Robert Petersen, and Dorothy Moore: *Alcohol, Tobacco, and Other Drugs May Harm the Newborn.* United States Department of Health and Human Services, Rockville, Maryland; 1990.

Cornelius, Llewellyn B.: Barriers to medical care for white, black, and Hispanic American children. *Journal of the National Medical Association*, 85(4):281–288; 1993.

Corporation for Public Broadcasting: *Miracle of Life.* Video production airing on public broadcasting series NOVA. Corporation for Public Broadcasting, Films for Humanities and Sciences, Monmouth Junction, New Jersey; 1983.

Craven, Ruth F.: *Fundamentals of Nursing*, 2nd edition. Lippincott–Raven Publishers, Philadelphia; 1996.

Cunningham, Gary, and Marshall Lindheimer: Hypertension in pregnancy. *New England Journal of Medicine*, 326(14):927–931; 1992.

Davis, Matthew, ed.: *Health Care Reform Update*, 1(8). National Association for Home Care; Washington D.C.; May 12, 1993.

Dingell, John D., and Committee of Conference: *Conference Report, ADAMNA Reorganization Act. Title V. Home Visiting Services for At-Risk Families.* 102nd Congress, 2nd Session, House of Representatives, Report 102-546. U.S. House of Representatives, Washington, D.C.; 1994.

Donar, Mary: Community care: Pediatric home mechanical ventilation. *Holistic Nursing Practice*, 2(2):68–80; 1988.

Falkner, F., ed.: *Prevention of Infant Mortality and Morbidity. Child Health and Development*, Volume 4. Karger, Basel, Switzerland; 1985.

Farber, Anne E.: *Survey of Home Visiting Programs for Children and Families in Pennsylvania, Executive Summary.* University of Pittsburgh, University Center for Social and Urban Reseach, Office of Child Development, Pittsburgh, Pennsylvania; 1996.

Fitzgerald, Susan: 1 in 6 New mothers used cocaine, study finds. *Philadelphia Inquirer*; April 8, 1989.

Fitzgerald, Susan: How three nations shape birth. *Philadelphia Inquirer, Suburban Edition*; April 27, 1993.

Friesen, Barbara J., Joanne Griesbach, Judith Jacobs, Judith Katz-Leavy, and Dennis Olson: Improving services for families. *Children Today*, pp. 18–22; July–August 1988.

Federal Register: Medicare regulations. *Federal Register: Rules and Regulations*, 54(153); August 14, 1989.

Fleming, Barbara W.: Assessing and promoting positive parenting in adolescent mothers. *MCN*, 18: 32–37; January–February 1993.

Grabert, B., C. Wardell, and S. Harburg: Home phototherapy. *Clinical Pediatrics*, 25:291–294; 1986.

Harrison, H., and A. Kositsky: *The Premature Baby Book*. St. Martin's Press, New York; 1983.

Henrikson, Mary, Ginna Wall, Dona Lethbridge, and Vicki McClurg: Nursing diagnosis and obstetric, gynecologic, and neonatal nursing: Breastfeeding as an example. *JOGN Thoughts and Opinions*, 21(6); November–December 1992.

Herman, Robin: France wants me to have this baby. *Washington Post*; May 1, 1990.

Hoerlin, Bettina Yaffe: *Targeting for the Future: Health Care in the Philadelphia Region*. Report to The Pew Charitable Trusts, Philadelphia, Pennsylvania; January 1989.

Howard, Tracy: *Kids Ending Hunger. What Can We Do?* Andrews and McMeel, A Universal Press Syndicate Co., Kansas City, Missouri; 1992.

Hyde-Robertson, Barbara L.: The necessity for maternal–infant perinatal home care. National Association for Home Care, Washington, D.C. *Caring*, pp. 26–31; December 1992.

Infante-Rivard, Claire, Gisele Filion, Mona Baumgarten, Madeleine Bourassa, Johanne Labelle, and Monique Messier: A public health home intervention among families of low socioeconomic status. *CHC*, 18(2):102; Spring 1989.

Institute of Medicine: *Nutrition During Pregnancy and Lactation*. National Academy Press, Washington, D.C.; 1990

Johns Hopkins Oral Rehydration Project: *Outpatient Oral Rehydration Therapy Protocol*. Johns Hopkins Oral Rehydration Project, Baltimore, Maryland; 1991.

Johnson, S., and D. Kraut: *Pregnancy and Bedrest: A Guide for the Pregnant Woman and Her Family*. St. Martin's Press, New York; 1990.

Langevin, Jeanne: Using home health aids in a high-risk infant program. *Caring*, pp. 40-43. National Association for Home Care, Washington, D.C.; June 1988.

Marecki, Marsha: Postpartum followup goals and assessment. *JOGN*, pp. 214–218; August 1979.

Marks, Margaret G.: *Introductory Pediatric Nursing*, 4th edition. Lippincott–Raven Publishers, Philadelphia; 1994.

McAnarney, Elizabeth R.: Experience with an adolescent health care program. *Public Health Reports*, 90(5):412–416; September–October 1975.

McAnarney, Elizabeth R.: Development of an adolescent maternity project in Rochester, New York. *Public Health Reports*, 92(2):154–159; March–April 1977.

NAACOG: *Criteria Established for Identifying At-Risk Infants*, 14(10). NAACOG, Washington, D.C.; October 1987.

NAACOG: *OGN Nursing Practice Resource: Neonatal Skin Care*. NAACOG, Washington, D.C.; 1992.

National Center for Education in Maternal and Child Health: *Reaching Out: A Directory of National Organizations Related to Maternal and Child Health*. National Center for Education in Maternal and Child Health, Washington, D.C.; March 1989.

Nettina, Sandra M.: *Lippincott Manual of Nursing Practice*, 6th edition. Lippincott–Raven Publishers, Philadelphia; 1996.

North Carolina Department of Health: *MCH Manual*. Department of Public Health, Durham, North Carolina; 1992.

Nuttal, P.: Maternal responses to home apnea monitoring of infants. *Nursing Research*, 37:354–357; 1988.

Oehler, Jerri N., et al.: How to target infants at highest risk for developmental delay. *Maternal-Child Nursing*, 18:20–23; January–February 1993.

Olds, D.: The prenatal/infancy project: A strategy for responding to the needs of high risk mothers and their children. *Prevention in Human Services*, 7(1):59–87; 1989.

Olds, D., C. Henderson, R. Tatlebaum, and R. Chamberlin: Improving the delivery of prenatal care and outcomes of pregnancy: A randomized trial of nurse home visitation. *Pediatrics*, 77(1):16–28; January 1986.

Olds, D., and H. Kitzman: Can home visitation improve the health of women and children at environmental risk? *Pediatrics*, 1(1):108–116; July 1990.

Pennsylvania Department of Health: *Block Grant, Commonwealth of Pennsylvania Preventive and Primary Care Services for Pregnant Women, Mothers, and Infants up to Age 1, Component A*, p. 64. Pennsylvania Department of Health, Division of Maternal Child Health, Harrisburg, Pennsylvania 1992.

Pennsylvania Department of Health: *Vital Statistics 1990*. Pennsylvania Department of Health, State Health Data Center, Harrisburg, Pennsylvania; 1992.

Pennsylvania Healthy Mothers, Healthy Babies Coalition: *Pennsylvania Healthy Mothers, Healthy Babies Coalition* Pennsylvania Healthy Mothers, Healthy Babies Coalition, Bryn Mawr, Pennsylvania 1992.

Pennsylvania Partnerships for Children: *Our Children, Our Future*. Breakfast on Children's Health Issues. Pennsylvania Partnerships for Children, Harrisburg, Pennsylvania; October 9, 1991.

Pennsylvania Partnerships for Children: *Kids Count*. State Grant Proposal for Pennsylvania. Pennsylvania Partnerships for Children, Harrisburg, Pennsylvania; August 13, 1992.

Perrin, James M.: Chronically ill children, in America, the case for home care. *Journal for Physicians in Home Care*; Spring 1987.

Philadelphia Department of Public Health: *Selected Resident Birth and Death Data by Health District, by Census Tract and by Neighborhood, 1983–1993*. Department of Public Health, Philadelphia; 1994.

Reece, S.: Social support and the early maternal experience for primiparas over 35. *Maternal–Child Nursing Journal*, 3:91–98; July–September 1993.

Reeder, S., L. Martin, and D. Koniak-Griffin: *Maternity Nursing, Family Newborn and Women's Health Care*, 18th edition. Lippincott–Raven Publishers, Philadelphia; 1997.

Richmond, Frederick, Martha Wade Steketee, et al.: *The State of the Child: A Profile of Pennsylvania's Children*. Waldman Graphics, Philadelphia; 1993.

Roberts, Joyce: Current perspectives in preeclampsia. *Journal of Nurse Midwifery*, 39(2):70–90; 1994.

Rogatz, Peter: Perspective on home care. *Public Health Nursing*, 4(1):7–8; March 1987.

Rosen, C., D. Glaze, and J. Frost: Home monitor followup of persistent apnea and bradycardia in preterm infants. *American Journal of Diseases in Children*, 140:547–550; 1986.

Shelton, Terri I., Elizabeth Jeppson, and Beverly Johnson: *Family Centered Care for Children with Special Health Care Needs*, 2nd edition. Association for the Care of Children's Health, U.S. Public Health Service, Division of Maternal Child Health, Rockville, Maryland; 1987.

Sills, Joanne: Infant deaths soar in areas. *Philadelphia Daily News*; July 8, 1992.

Sirkka, L.: Health promotion in child and family health care: The role of the Finnish public health nurses. *Public Health Nursing*, 11(1):32–37; February 1994.

Smith, Judy: The dangers of prenatal cocaine use. *Maternal-Child Nursing*, 13:174–179; May–June 1992.

South Carolina Department of Health and Environmental Control: *Comprehensive Risk Screening for Patient Referrals*. South Carolina Department of Health and Environmental Control, Maternal Health, Columbia, South Carolina; October 1992.

Stanwick, Richard S., Michael E. K. Moffat, Yvonne Robitaille, Aline Edmond, and Caroline Dok: An evaluation of the routine postnatal public health nurse home visit. *Canadian Journal of Public Health,* 73:200–205; May–June 1982.

Starn, J.: Community health nursing visits for at risk women and infants. *Journal of Community Health Nursing,* 9(2):103–110; 1992.

Streeter, N. S.: Discharge planning home care. *Journal of Perinatal and Neonatal Nursing* 5(1); 1991.

Sullivan, Joan, et al.: Can we help the substance abusing mother and infant? *Maternal-Child Nursing,* 18:153–157; May–June 1993.

United Way of Pennsylvania: *Report of the Success-By-Six Coalition: Helping All Children Succeed for Life.* United Way of Pennsylvania, Harrisburg, Pennsylvania; June 1992.

U.S.D.L., Occupational Safety and Health, Office of Health Compliance Assistance: *OSHA Instruction CPL 2-2, 44A,* p. 4. U.S. Department of Labor Occupational Safety and Health, Office of Health Compliance Assistance, Washington, D.C.; August 15, 1988.

U.S.D.P.H., Agency for Health Care Policy and Research: *The 50 Most Frequent Diagnosis-Related Groups (DRO's), Diagnoses, and Procedures: Statistics by Hospital Size and Location.* Hospital Studies Program Research Note 13. U.S. Department of Public Health, Agency for Health Care Policy and Research, Rockville, Maryland; September 1990.

U.S.D.P.H., Agency for Health Care Policy and Research: *Research Activities: Contracts Awarded for Low Birthweight, Health Care for Women, Barriers to Quality Care Persist.* Publication No. 158. U.S. Department of Public Health, Agency for Health Care Policy and Research, Rockville, Maryland; November 1992.

U.S.D.P.H., Agency for Health Care Policy and Research: *Research Activities: Number of Uninsured Children on the Rise, Less than 15 Percent of America's Health Care Dollar Spent on Children.* Publication No. 162. U.S. Department of Public Health, Agency for Health Care Policy and Research, Rockville, Maryland; March 1993.

U.S.D.P.H., Agency for Health Care Policy and Research: *Research Activities: Women Planning Pregnancy Often Switch to HMO's.* Publication No. 163. U.S. Department of Public Health, Agency for Health Care Policy and Research, Rockville, Maryland; April 1993.

U.S.D.P.H., Agency for Health Care Policy and Research: *Research Activities: Uninsured Patients More Likely to Die Prematurely.* Publication No. 169. U.S. Department of Public Health, Agency for Health Care Policy and Research, Rockville, Maryland; October 1993.

U.S.D.P.H., Agency for Health Care Policy and Research: *Research Activities: Financially Troubled Hospitals Face Difficult Choices, Outlook Poor for Very Young Babies with AIDS, Teen Health Programs Often Deficient in On Site Services.* Publication No. 170. U.S. Department of Public Health, Agency for Health Care Policy and Research, Rockville, Maryland; November 1993.

U.S.D.P.H.H.S.: *Caring for Our Future: The Content of Prenatal Care.* U.S. Department of Public Health and Human Services, Washington, D.C.; 1989.

Vrazo, Fawn: Pregnant doctors in distress. *Philadeinhia Inquirer;* February 17, 1990.

Vrazo, Fawn: Lying in is now out for many new mothers. *Philadelphia Inquirer;* August 17, 1990.

Vrazo, Fawn: Lying in is out as insurers cut post-childbirth coverage. *Philadelphia Inquirer;* August 7, 1993.

Wasik, B., D. Bryant, and C. Lyons: *Home Visiting: Procedures for Helping Families.* Sage Publications, Newbury Park, California; 1990.

Weston, Donna R., Barbara Ivins, Barry Zuckerman, Coryl Jones, and Richard Lopez: *Drug Exposed Babies: Research and Clinical Issues.* DC(S). National Center for Clinical Infant Programs, Washington, D.C.; June 1989.

Williams, Lenore, and Mary Cooper: Nurse managed postpartum home care. *JOGN Principles and Practice,* pp. 25–31; January–February 1993.

Wisconsin Association for Perinatal Care: *Early Discharge—Short Term Length of Stay.* Wisconsin Association for Perinatal Care; June 1993.

Yariover, Mark J., Deloras Jones, and Michael D. Miller: Perinatal care of low risk mothers and infants. *New England Journal of Medicine*, 294(13):702–705; March 25, 1976.

Young, L., D. Creighton, and R. Sauve: The needs of families of infants discharged home with continous oxygen therapy. *Journal of Obstetric, Gynecolgic, and Neonatal Nursing*, 17:187–193; 1987.

Zuravin, Susan J.: *Child Maltreatment and Teenage First Births: A Relationship Mediated by Chronic Sociodemographic Stress?* American Orthopsychiatric Association; January 1988.

Additional Resources

Free or low-cost educational material can be obtained from the following additional health information resources.

U.S. Department of Health and Human Services

Public Health Service Office of Disease Prevention and Health Promotion

ONHIC, P.O. Box 1133

Washington, DC 20013-1133

(800) 336-4797

Request the *Health Information Resources Catalogue*

Maternal Child Health Bureau

March of Dimes Birth Defects Foundation

National Center for Education in Maternal Child Health

Write to: National Maternal Child Health Clearing House

8201 Greensboro Drive, Suite 600

McLean, VA 22102

(703) 821-8955, ext. 254 or 265

Request *Prenatal Care, A Resource Guide*

Danger Signs

Danger Signs	**Potential Problem**
1. Vaginal bleeding, no matter how slight (not pink show at term); significant if before 37 weeks	Placenta previa, abruptio placenta, danger of loss of oxygen to fetus, premature delivery
2. Swelling face or fingers	Hypertension, eclamptic crisis
3. Severe continuous headaches	Hypertension, eclamptic crisis
4. Dimness, blurring of vision, flashes of light or dots before eyes	Hypertension, eclamptic crisis
5. Abdominal pain	Abruptio placenta
6. Persistent vomiting	Hypertensive, eclamptic crisis, or dehydration that could cause premature labor
7. Fever, chills, pain urinating, or foul-smelling vaginal discharge	Infection
8. Sudden escape of fluid from vagina	Rupture of membranes before 37 weeks, causing premature labor
9. Sudden decrease or absence of fetal movement over 24 hours	Fetal compromise
10. Regular, uterine contractions before 37 weeks	Premature labor

THE PRENATAL DATA COLLECTION AND RISK SCORING TOOL

ANTEPARTUM RISK SCORING INDEX

Patient's Name ____

Address ____

Phone number _______________________ Insurance company _______________________

OB care provider _______________________ Phone number _______________________

Gestational date _______________________ Today's date _______________________

A score of 10 or more on this index indicates a client is at high risk.
However, in assessing your future course of action with each client, look at absolute scores instead of just the designation of low or high risk. For example, the diabetic client with no other problems rates 10 points and therefore is considered at high risk. However, the obese patient (5) who has a drinking problem (5) and is a heavy smoker (5) scores 15 points; she may be at still greater risk.

Scoring Value	Condition	Actual Score of Client
Anatomical Abnormalities		
10	Uterine malformation	( )
10	Incompetent cervix	( )
10	Abnormal fetal position	( )
10	Hydramnios	( )
5	Clinically small pelvis	( )
10	Multiple pregnancy	( )
10	Vaginal spotting	( )
Miscellaneous (this pregnancy)		
5	Age 15	( )
5	Age 35	( )
5	Weight 100 lbs.	( )
5	Weight 200 lbs.	( )
1	Mild anemia, 9.0–10.9 hemoglobin	( )
5	Severe anemia, 9.0 hemoglobin	( )
10	Sickle cell disease or trait	( )
5	Rh sensitized, first time	( )
5	Positive serology	( )
5	Positive PPD	( )
3	Viral disease	( )
3	Flu syndrome	( )

(continued)

Scoring Value	Condition	Actual Score of Client
Miscellaneous (this pregnancy)		
3	Vaginitis	( )
5	Abnormal cervical cytology	( )
10	Pulmonary dysfunction	( )
10	Post-term (over 42 wk)	( )
10	Intrauterine growth retardation	( )
5	Emotional problems	( )
5	Smoking	( )
5	Alcohol abuse	( )
5	Excessive drug use, nonnarcotic	( )
10	Narcotic use	( )
10	No-care client (no previous medical care until late in pregnancy)	( )
Cardiovascular Disorders		
10	Class I heart disease	( )
10	Severe heart disease, classes (II–IV)	( )
10	Chronic hypertension	( )
3	History of preeclampsia	( )
5	History of eclampsia	( )
5	Mild preeclampsia	( )
10	Moderate–severe preeclampsia	( )
Renal Disorders		
5	History of GU infection (including acute cystitis)	( )
10	Acute pyelonephritis	( )
10	Moderate–severe renal disease	( )
Metabolic Disorders		
3	Family history of diabetes	( )
5	Diabetes (Type II, III, IV)	( )
10	Diabetes (Type I)	( )
5	Thyroid disease	( )
3	Previous endocrine ablation	( )
History		
3	Therapeutic abortion	( )
5	Habitual abortion	( )
10	Previous stillbirth	( )
10	Previous low birth weight infant	( )
10	Previous neonatal death	( )
5	Previous infant >10 lbs	( )
3	Previous cesarean section	( )
1	Rh neg., nonsensitized	( )
10	Rh neg., sensitized	( )
5	Multiparity >5	( )
5	Epilepsy	( )
5	Previous fetal anomalies	( )
3	Drug allergy	( )

Prenatal Universal Home Risk Assessment

Prenatal Universal Home Risk Assessment

Mother's Name ____ D.O.B _______________

Address _________________________ City ___________ Zip _________ Phone: _____________

Emergency contact ____ Phone: _____________

Language ________________ Race _____ Marital status _________ Education ______________ Occupation _______________

Gravida _____ Para _____   LMP / /   EDC / /   Wks. gest. _____

Is patient enrolled in insurance plan?   Yes ( ) No ( )   Ins. type _____________________

Has patient notified caseworker of pregnancy?   Yes ( ) No ( )   Ins. # _______________________

Has patient been informed of insurance benefits MA/HMO?   Yes ( ) No ( )   Mother SS #: ________________

Current medications ________________________________   Hosp. of delivery ________________

MOTHER ASSESSMENT		NORM	ABNORMAL F/U M.D.	ABNORMAL F/U Home Care provider	COMMENTS
Skin					
Metabolic (TPR)					
Neuro					
HEENT					
CardioVasc. Chest	BP Lungs/Breasts				
Musculoskeletal	Upper/Lower Ext.				
GI	Nutrition/Elimin.				
GU	Voiding/Eval. of Lochia				

MEDICAL HISTORY	p - past c - current	F/U M.D.	F/U Home Care provider	COMMENTS
1. Congenital anomalies				
2. Genetic diseases				
3. Multiple births				
4. Diabetes melitus, gest. diab.				
5. Hypertension; PIH				
6. Heart, pulmonary dis.				
7. Urinary tract probs.				
8. IUGR; Low birth weight				
9. Placenta previa, abruption				
10. Phlebitis, varicosities				
11. Convulsive disorder				
12. Anemia, hemoglobinopathy				
13. PROM, premature labor				
14. Venereal disease				
15. HBV; HIV+, AIDS				
16. Other				

Patient name: ____

NUTRITION ASSESSMENT

Pre-pregnancy wt. ______ wt. gain to date _______ goal for wt. gain _________ Previous dietary therapy_______________

Medical/Psychosocial factors affecting diet ____

Adequate Resources for _______ cooking _______ shopping ________ food storage. Environment free of insects yes ( ) no ( ) rodents yes ( ) no ( )

Dietary recall (24 hrs.)____ Knowledge of nutrition

(circle risk score if applicable)

I. Life Transitions
2 denial/rejection re: pregnancy
1 Hx current/recent incest/rape victim
1 Hx infant/child chronic disability
1 Hx of fetal death/other inf./preg.loss
1 adoption/termination considered
1 suspected domestic violence

II. Emotional Status
1 Hx of mental illness/mental health treat./hosp.
1 unresolved grief/signif. loss
2 suicidal ideation
1 feels isolation/alone/inadeq. support system
1 questionable coping
1 Hx of postpartum depression
1 evidence of low self-esteem

III. Substance Abuse/Risk-Taking Behaviors
3 current/recent abuse or ETOH
3 current/recent abuse of street drugs
3 current/recent abuse of presc. meds
1 law enforcement involvement
1 sexual risk-taking behaviors
1 tobacco use or 2nd-hand smoke exposure

IV. Parenting issues (observed/expressed)
1 teen/inexperienced parent
1 develop. issues (child/fam. expectations)
1 discipline issues
1 relationship issues (bond/nurturing)
1 hx child abuse/neglect, now resolved
2 child abuse/neglect, current
1 3 or more children< 6 yrs. of age

V. Educational/Cultural Factors
1 low literacy/limited intellectual ability
1 language barriers
1 cognitve deficits
1 ed. level 12th or <
2 ed. level 10th or <
3 ed. level 9th or < or < 17 y.o.
1 Culture/beliefs

VI. Economic/Resource Needs
1 insuff. income to meet basic needs
1 no transportation
2 inadequate food
1 legal needs
2 chronic difficulty accessing "system"
1 child care problems
1 Medicaid problems

VII. Maternal Medical/Nutrition Factors
2 abnl. phys. fndgs. this assess.
1 probs. w/ chosen FP method
1 short interconceptual period (< 1 yr.)
1 grand multigravid (> 7 preg.)
2 anemia mother <10.8
2 chronic disease
3 HIV+/AIDS
1 prob. initiating breastfeeding
1 pica
1 anorexia/bulemia/fad diets
3 inadequate prenatal care
3 previous PTB, LBW, IUGR

VIII. Environmental
1 housing
1 utilities
1 water/sewer
1 refrigeration
1 high risk/unsafe neighborhood
1 inadeq. prep. for infant

SUMMARY OF ASSESSMENT AND RISK FACTORS

____

____

REFERRALS/PLAN Prenatal Visit	DATE OF APPT.	CONTACT PERSON/PROVIDER	PHONE
WIC			
Nutritionist			
Social Worker			
M.A. Caseworker			
Other			

EVALUATION
____ Discharge to Primary, no further HC required.   PCP name:_______________________
____ Open to Home Care follow-up   Address: _______________________

NRSG INTERVENTIONS/TEACHING	DONE	DEFERRED TO HC	EVALUATION (response to teaching)
Prenatal Care			
Nutrition			
Childbirth Education			
Infection Control/Safety			
Breastfeeding			
S/S Pregnancy Complications			

Nurse signature _________________________________ date _________________

Guidelines for Completion of Home Health Certification and Plan of Treatment

These guidelines are intended to clarify certain fields on the HCFA 485 form. **IT IS ESSENTIAL THAT ALL INFORMATION BE CURRENT AND THAT NO BLANKS ARE LEFT,** except as specified below.

1. Patient HI claim—the health insurance number
2. SOC date—the start of care date (ie, date of first visit for this home care admission)
3. Certification period—

The *initial certification period* (62 days) begins on the start of care date. For example, if the start of care is 10/01/93, the POC is generated 10/01/93. The certification period would be 10/01/93 to 12/01/93. A recertification Plan of Care (POC) must be generated and signed by the physician *before* the initial or previous certification period expires. In the example above, the recertification POC must be completed and signed by the physician before 12/02/93. The next recertification period would be 12/02/93 to 02/02/93.

4. Medical record no.—leave blank
5. Provider no.—leave blank
6. Patient name and address—self-explanatory
7. Provider's name and address—Name and address of home care agency.
8. Date of birth—client's date of birth
9. Sex—client's sex
10. Medications—specify medication, dose (include the concentration), route, frequency. *Verify current medication orders on day of discharge.*
11. Diagnosis—the primary diagnosis and ICD-9 Code; date of onset
12. Surgical procedure and date—indicate type of surgery and date or write "N/A."
13. Other pertinent diagnosis—the secondary diagnosis, if applicable, ICD-9 code; date of onset
14. Durable medical equipment and supplies—for example: IV pole, pump, and "related disposal supplies" (individual disposables do not have to be listed).
15. Safety Measures—indicate the safety precautions to be observed or taught *related to the type of care provided.* For example: sharps container, for IV therapy patients; reflux precautions, for child with reflux; C-R monitor alarm limits, for patients on a monitor; three-prong (grounded) plugs for equipment; "toddler proofing" medications and supplies. In other words, describe any safety measure needed because of client's condition or functional limitation. For clients on service for health supervision such as the Episcopal high-risk patients, include "911, universal precautions, basic home safety for infant/toddler," *and anything else the nurse observes in the home* related to safety.
16. Nutritional requirements—specify type of diet or formula type, amount, frequency, and route.
17. Allergies or no known allergies (NKA) should be documented.
18A. Functional limitations—self-explanatory. If infant, check "other" and write "infant."
18B. Activity permitted—check any that apply; if infant, check "other" and write "infant."
19. Mental status—check any that apply; if infant, check "other" and write "infant."
20. Prognosis—as per the nurse's judgment; check one.
21. Orders for discipline and treatments—specify the *discipline frequency* and *duration;* for example, skilled nursing 3×/week × 2 weeks, then D/C (or then reevaluate); HHA 8 hr/day, 5×/week × 8 weeks.

    For treatment orders, write *specifics.* For example, assess wound and caregiver's ability to perform dressing change; assess caregiver's ability to administer medications; chest physical therapy with suction every 3 hours or as needed; weekly laboratory tests to include complete blood count with differential and platelets.

    Orders for patients who are part of the High Risk Follow-up Program are written as follows:
    Initial certification (first 62 days of service)

SN (skilled nursing) visits:

1. (3-unit)* evaluation on _________ followed by:
3. (2-unit)* × 1 week (within 7-10 days of SOC)
2. (2-unit)* × 2 weeks
1. (2-unit)* × 5–6 weeks (not to exceed 15 units in last 30 days of certification period.

Provide: Infant history and physical assessment, evaluation, and plan of care; weights and measurements; assessment of growth and development; compliance with appointments; nutritional teaching; parenting education; link with community resources as needed.

Identify: Barriers to care and parenting problems. Initiate resolution and referrals as needed.

First recertification (2nd 62 days)

Skilled Nursing Visits:

1 (2-unit)* skilled nursing visit 2×/month for 8 weeks (not to exceed 15 units per 30 days) to provide:

Infant physical assessment, weights, and measurements; assessment of growth and development; assessment of caregiver's compliance with appointments; nutritional support and teaching; parenting education; follow-up with community resource linkages as needed.

Second recertification (3rd 62 days)

Skilled Nursing Visits:

1 (2-unit)* visit 1×/month for 8 weeks

Provide: Infant physical assessment, weights, and measurements; assessment of growth and development; assessment of caregiver's compliance with appointments; nutritional support and teaching; parenting education; follow-up with community resource linkages as needed.

22. Goals/rehabilitation potential/discharge plans—goals must be specific and measurable; for example, wound will heal without complication, caregiver(s) will be independent in dressing change and medication administration, infant will gain weight, patient will maintain O_2 saturations greater than 94% SAO_2. Rehabilitation potential applies only to clients receiving physical therapy, speech therapy, or occupational therapy. Discharge plans must be specific and include a timeframe.

23. Verbal start of care date and nurse's signature and date where applicable—date of start of care (ie, first visit).

24. Physician's name and address—self-explanatory.

25. Date home health agency received signed plan of care—leave blank.

26. Initial orders or recertification should be checked as applicable.

The following are important state regulations:

The Initial Plan of Care should be generated and mailed to the attending physician for countersignature within 48 hours of the first visit. **The signed original must be returned from the physician and incorporated into the medical record within 21 days of the start of care.**

The Recertification Plan of Care should be generated and mailed to the physician for countersignature 14 days before the expiration date of the previous POC. **The signed original must be signed by the physician, returned to the office, and incorporated into the medical record within 62 days of the previous POC** (by the time the previous POC expires).

Home Health Certification and Plan of Treatment

Department of Health and Human Services
Health Care Financing Administration

Form Approved
OMB No. 0938-0357

HOME HEALTH CERTIFICATION AND PLAN OF TREATMENT

1. Patient's HI Claim No.	2. SOC Date	3. Certification Period From: To:	4. Medical Record No.	5. Provider No.

6. Patient's Name and Address	7. Provider's Name and Address.

8. Date of Birth:	9. Sex [ ] M [ ] F	10. Medications: Dose/Frequency/Route (N)ew (C)hanged

11. ICD-9-CM	Principal Diagnosis	Date

12. ICD-9-CM	Surgical Procedure	Date

13. ICD-9-CM	Other Pertinent Diagnoses	Date

14. DME and Supplies	15. Safety Measures:

16. Nutritional Req.	17. Allergies:

18.A. Functional Limitations

1	[ ] Amputation	5	[ ] Paralysis	9	[ ] Legally Blind
2	[ ] Bowel/Bladder (Incontinence)	6	[ ] Endurance	A	[ ] Dyspnea With Minimal Exertion
3	[ ] Contracture	7	[ ] Ambulation	B	[ ] Other (Specify)
4	[ ] Hearing	8	[ ] Speech		

18.B. Activities Permitted

1	[ ] Complete Bedrest	6	[ ] Partial Weight Bearing	A	[ ] Wheelchair
2	[ ] Bedrest BRP	7	[ ] Independent At Home	B	[ ] Walker
3	[ ] Up As Tolerated	8	[ ] Crutches	C	[ ] No Restrictions
4	[ ] Transfer Bed/Chair	9	[ ] Cane	D	[ ] Other (Specify)
5	[ ] Exercises Prescribed				

19. Mental Status:	1	[ ] Oriented	3	[ ] Forgetful	5	[ ] Disoriented	7	[ ] Agitated
	2	[ ] Comatose	4	[ ] Depressed	6	[ ] Lethargic	8	[ ] Other

20. Prognosis:	1	[ ] Poor	2	[ ] Guarded	3	[ ] Fair	4	[ ] Good	5	[ ] Excellent

21. Orders for Discipline and Treatments (Specify Amount/Frequency/Duration)

Individualized if needed for

follow-up after initial assessment.

22. Goals/Rehabilitation Potential/Discharge Plans

23. Verbal Start of Care and Nurse's
Signature and Date Where Applicable:

24. Physician's Name and Address	25. Date HHA Received Signed POT	26. I [ ] certify [ ] recertify that the above home health services are required and are authorized by me with a written plan for treatment which will be periodically reviewed by me. This patient is under my care, is confined to his home, and is in need of intermittent skilled nursing care and/or physical or speech therapy or has been furnished home health services based on such a need and no longer has a need for such care or therapy, but continues to need occupational therapy.
27. Attending Physician's Signature (Required on 485 Kept on File in Medical Records of HHA)	Date Signed	

Form HCFA-485 (U4) (4-87)

Consent for Treatment, Release of Information, Assignment of Benefits, Notice of Client Rights

Client Name: ____

Address: ____

City: ________________ State: __________ Zip: ___________ Phone: (___)____________

Insurance Company:_________________________________ Insurance I.D.#

I, the _________________________ (of the patient), intending to be legally bound, hereby:

1. Consent to such care and treatment by ___________________, and its employees and agents (collectively, the "Agency"), as prescribed by the client's physician or dictated by the client's condition.

2. Authorize the Agency to release any medical records in its possession concerning the client as may be required by law or to pay benefits on the client's behalf. I authorize the client's physicians, insurors, and hospitals to release such medical records to the Agency at the Agency's request.

3. Authorize my insuror to disclose to the Agency the terms and extent of my coverage, and the amount of payments made to me for services provided by the Agency.

4. Assign, transfer and set over to the Agency all of my or the client's rights to insurance proceeds or other funds to which I am or the patient is or will become entitled as a result of the services rendered by the Agency.

5. Consent to and authorize payment, which would otherwise be payable to me or the client, to be made directly to the Agency. The Agency may issue a receipt for such payment which shall discharge the insurance company of its obligations under the policy to the extent of such payment.

6. Agree that I remain individually responsible to pay the Agency for all charges not paid for any reason by the insurer or other third-party payor. I understand that payment in full is due upon receipt of my bill. If payment for the Agency's service is made directly to me by my insuror, I agree to endorse the check to ___________________ and forward it to the Agency within three days of receipt.

A photocopy of this document, if executed, shall be considered as effective and valid as the original.

The effect of this form and the Client's Rights and Responsibilities on the back of this form have been explained to me by the Agency and I understand its content and significance.

Date: _____________________ Signature: _________________________________

Name: _________________________________

(Please Print)

Home Health Care Client's Bill of Rights/Responsibilities

As a home health care client you have the right to:

1. Be given information about your rights and responsibilities for receiving home health care services, in terms and language you can reasonably expect to understand.

2. Receive a timely response from the Home Health Care Agency regarding your request for home health care services.

3. Be given information of the Home Health Care Agency charges and policy concerning payment for services, including your eligibility for third party reimbursement.

4. Choose your home health care providers.

5. Be given appropriate and professional quality home health care services without discrimination against your race, creed, color, religion, sex, national origin, sexual preference, handicap, or age.

6. Be treated with courtesy and respect by all who provide home health care services to you; to have your property treated with respect.

7. Be given proper identification by name and title of everyone who provides home health care services to you.

8. Be given the necessary information so you will be able to give informed consent for your treatment before the start of any treatment.

9. Participate in the development of your home health care plan, to be informed in advance about the care to be provided and any changes in the care to be provided, including anticipated transfer of your care to another health care facility and/or termination of home health care services.

10. To be advised in advance of the disciplines that will provide care, and the frequency of visits proposed to be provided.

11. Be given data privacy and confidentiality; review your clinical record at your request.

12. Voice grievances regarding treatment or care that is (or fails to be) furnished, or regarding any lack of respect for privacy by anyone who is furnishing services on behalf of the home health care agency, without being subject to discrimination or reprisal for doing so.

    - Call to voice a grievance and/or recommend changes in policies or services.
    - Medicare/Medicaid clients may also call a Hotline # (1-800-222-0989) to report grievances from 8: 30 AM-5:00 PM with answering service for nonbusiness hours. This is *not* the number to reach the Home Health Care Agency or to obtain Medicare coverage/billing information.

13. Refuse all or part of your care to the extent permitted by law; to be informed of the expected consequences of such action.

Nursing Plan of Care and Progress Record

Nursing Plan of Care and Progress Record

Client Name: ____ __

Address: ____

____

____

Phone: (__) ____________________________________

Allergies: ____

<u>Immunization Status</u>

1. Did infant receive any immunizations at last visit?　　yes　　no

2. Has infant received any immunizations since birth?　　yes　　no

3. If yes, when and which ones? (if changed from last visit) __________ Name of last pediatric provider: ______________________

4. Is infant appropriately immunized? (as reported by caregiver)　　yes　　no

5. If no, why? (as explained by caregiver) _________________________ Date of last appt. ________________________

	Yes	No
HHA Supervisory Visit	☐ Yes	☐ No
PT satisfied with care?	☐ Yes	☐ No
HHA following care plan?	☐ Yes	☐ No
Care plan updated?	☐ Yes	☐ No
HHA's name		

Lead Screening Status

1. Is infant the appropriate age for lead screening?　　yes　　no
2. If yes, does caregiver know if it was done?　　yes　　no
3. Does caregiver know results?　　yes　　no

Date of next appt. ________________________

Skilled Observation/Assessment

	Normal	Abnormal	Describe		Normal	Abnormal	Describe
Metabolic (TPR)				Genitourinary			
HEENT				Musculoskeletal			
Cardiovascular				Neurologic			
Respiratory				Integumentary			
ABD/G.I.				Psychosocial			
Nutrition/Wt.				Other			

Medical Diagnosis ____

Reason for Visit/Homecare Needs ____

Nursing Diagnosis(es) ____

Short-Term Goal(s) ____

Long-Term Goal(s) ____

Nursing Interventions (treatment, teaching, etc.) ____

____

____

____

Evaluation (response to interventions) ____

____

____

____

Date and Nursing Care Plan for next visit ____

____

Communication to M.D./Agency Office/Other ____

Charge in orders/Change in medication ____

(specify change and attach completed verbal order form)

RN Signature: ___________________________ License #: _______________________ Date: ___________________

Discharge Summary

Patient Name: _________________________   Insurance: _________________________

Diagnosis: _________________________   I.D. #: _________________________

Date of first visit: _________   Date of discharge visit: _________   Client/Caregiver notified: ☐ Yes ☐ No

Number of visits: RN _____ LPN _____ PT _____ OT _____ ST _____ Other: _________________________

(type of service)

Initiation of discharge: Physician (give name) _________________________ Date notified: _________

Physician's address _________________________

____

Reason for termination of service: ☐ Goals Met ☐ Noncompliance ☐ Transferred ☐ Refused Visit
☐ Re-Hospitalized ☐ Moved Out of Service Area ☐ Expired
☐ Placed/Adopted ☐ Insurance Changed/Denied ☐ Unable to Locate

Status of problems identified at admission and subsequently: _________________________

____

____

Overall status of client/family: _________________________

____

____

Summary of the care or service provided: _________________________

____

____

Referrals made and instructions given: _________________________

____

____

____

Disposition: ☐ Home   ☐ Hospital   ☐ Rehab   ☐ Hospice   ☐ Extended Care Facility

Name of organization to which client is being transferred (if applicable): _________________________

Nurse signature: _________________________   Date: _________

Physician signature: _________________________   Date: _________

(if required)

White's Classification of Diabetes in Pregnancy

Class A—Chemical diabetes (abnormal glucose tolerance test)
Class B—Maturity onset (age 20 years or older); duration under 10 years, no vascular lesions
Class C1—Age 10 to 19 years at onset
Class C2—10 to 19 years' duration
Class D1—Younger than 10 years at onset
Class D2—Over 20 years' duration
Class D3—Benign retinopathy
Class D4—Calcified vessels of legs
Class D5—Hypertension
Class E—No longer sought
Class F—Nephropathy
Class G—Many failures
Class H—Cardiopathy
Class R—Proliferative retinopathy
Class T—Renal transplant (added by Tagatz and colleagues of the University of Minnesota)

Perinatal Home Needs Assessment Tool

Client Data

Client's name _______________________

Nickname _______________________

Client's DOB __/__/__   Client's Age _____

Client's ins. type & no. _______________

Client's SS no. _______________________

Client's race ___ White ___ Black

___ Hispanic ___ Other

EDC _____ Weeks gestation ___________

Primary language _____________________

___ Home ___ Shelter ___ Homeless

___ Staying with relatives

Current residence address:

____
Street

____
City   Zip

Phone _______________________

Best time to contact _______________

Diagnoses

1. _______________________

2. _______________________

3. _______________________

Exacerbating potentials:

Emergency Contact Person/s

Name _______________________
                                        Age

Relationship _______________________

Phone _______________________

Address _______________________
              Street

____
City   Zip

Doctor (must use PCP if applicable)

Name _______________________

Hospital _______________________

Phone _______________________

Address _______________________
              Street

____
City   Zip

Consulting Doctors on Care

Phone _______________________

1. _______________________

2. _______________________

3. _______________________

Other consultants:

1. SW _______________________

2. other _______________________

____

1. Planned hospital for delivery _______________________

2. History of prenatal care this pregnancy _______________________

3. Planned delivery:

     Vaginal   C-section

____

I. Prior OB history: G _________ P _________

PIH _________ GDM _________ IDDM _________ Eclampsia _________

No. of children living with her, and their ages: _________________________________

____

Any children in foster care, or living elsewhere: _________________________________

____

____

II. Current State of Health:
1. Physical
2. Mental
3. Emotional
4. Social
5. Hospitalizations/Surgeries
6. Diet/Nutrition/weight prior to pregnancy; weight gain so far
7. Activity
8. Physical limitations
9. Support systems
10. Limitations
11. Medications—Time, Frequency, Amount, Purpose, Side effects

12. Teaching Needed

___ Transportation   ___ Self-treatment

___ Changes during pregnancy

___ Nutrition   ___ Home Safety   ___ Community Resources

         ___ utilities

         ___ phone

         ___ housing

         ___ cooking

         ___ water

         ___ respite

         ___ ref.

         ___ others

___ Growth/Dev.

___ Parenting Education

___ Budgeting of financial resources

___ Parenting skills   ___ Parenting education

___ Gestational diabetes   ___ Premature labor

___ Rupture of membranes   ___ Signs/Symptoms of Labor

13. Referrals already made: _________________________________

14. Referrals needed: _________________________________

___ WIC   ___ Wheels

____

IV. Family Data/Support Network:
  1. Other household members (name, age, medical issues)
  2. Other significant others/extended family members
      Are they available to assist with care of child—when delivered?
  3. Summary of household function—Do people work together?
      Do they get along? Who is in charge?
  4. Evidence of drug/ETOH use
  5. Smoker

Housing Information
1. Current residence __ Permanent __ Temporary

2. Type of residence __ House __ Apt. __ Shelter __ Other explain _______________________

3. Length of time in current residence ____

4. Are there Plans to Move? __ Yes __ No __ When? ____________________________

   New Address: ____

5. Layout of House:

   no. of bedrooms _______ no. of bathrooms ______

   __ Kitchen __ Dining area __ Living area __ Furniture

   Condition of House: ____

   Safety Issues at House:

   Outlets: __ 2 Prong __ 3 Prong __ Adeq. nos.
   __ Inadeq. nos.

   Smoke alarms: __ Yes __ No no. of alarms: _______________________________

   Stable railings: __ Yes __ No

   Adequate lighting: __ Yes __ No (specify)

   Emergency nos. Posted: __ Yes __ No

   Sanitation: no. of Bathrooms: __

   A. Is kitchen sanitary? __ Yes __ No (specify)

   B. Pest Control: Are the following present:

      __ Roaches __ Rats/Mice __ Flies

   C. Plumbing problems ____

      Medication storage: Specify plan for storage, if refrigeration needed

      Infection control needs surrounding care:

      Summary of client home needs assessment

   ____

   Problem list—Preliminary

   ____

   Plan

Forms Index and Explanation

1. **Prenatal Data Collection and Risk Scoring Tool (Appendix B)**

   Used to record risk factors provided by OB care provider and other medical-social sources. Additional data found at initial home evaluation should also be added to determine effect on high-risk scoring in assessing overall pregnancy risks.

2. **Prenatal Universal Home Risk Assessment Tool (Appendix C)**

   This record is used at the initial home evaluation and is completed by the nurse. Levels of care are assigned, based on levels of risk noted as 1s, 2s, and 3s on form. These correlate with a level of risk assignment found in the directions in the chapter on standards for risk categories.

3. **Instructions for completing Home Health Certification and Plan of Treatment from the Health Care Financing Administration (Appendices D and E).**

4. **Consent for Treatment, Release of Information, Assignment of Benefits, Notice of Client Rights form (Appendix F)**

   Required by federal certification and other organizations such as the National League for Nursing forms index or the Joint Commission for the Accreditation of Health Care Organizations.

5. **Nursing Plan of Care and Progress Record (Appendix H)**

   The standard record completed by the nurse for each visit after the initial visit.

6. **Discharge Summary (Appendix I)**

   To be completed by the nurse at the time of client discharge.

7. **Perinatal Home Needs Assessment Tool (Appendix K)**

   This is a supplemental form to the initial home risk assessment that provides more detail into socioeconomic difficulties the client may be facing. This provides the nurse with more detailed information that may be helpful in developing a nursing care plan for overall interventions. The form may be completed over the course of several visits.

Common Abbreviations in Maternal-Child Nursing

ABC	alternative birthing center; airway, breathing, circulation
AC	abdominal circumference
ADA	American Diabetes Association
ADL	activities of daily living
AFP	alpha-fetoprotein
AFV	amniotic fluid volume
AGA	average for gestational age
AIDS	acquired immune deficiency syndrome
AROM	artificial rupture of membranes
BAT	brown adipose tissue (brown fat)
BGS	blood glucose sample
BL	baseline (fetal heart rate baseline)
BMR	basal metabolic rate
BOW	bag of waters
BP	blood pressure
BPD	biparietal diameter; bronchopulmonary dysplasia
BPM	beats per minute
BSE	breast self-examination
BUN	blood urea nitrogen
CC	chest circumference; cord compression; chief complaint
cc	cubic centimeter
CDC	Centers for Disease Control
CHF	congestive heart failure
CID	cytomegalic inclusion disease
CMV	cytomegalovirus
cm	centimeter
CNM	certified nurse-midwife
CNS	central nervous system
CPAP	continuous positive airway pressure
CPD	cephalopelvic disproportion; citrate-phosphate-dextrose
CPR	cardiopulmonary resuscitation
C/S	cesarean section or c-section
DHS	Department of Health Services
dil	dilatation
D&C	dilatation and curettage

DES	diethylstilbestrol
DFMR	daily fetal movement response
DM	diabetes mellitus
DOB	date of birth
DRG	diagnostic related groups
DTR	deep tendon reflexes
ECMO	extracorporeal membrane oxygenator
EDC	estimated date or confinement
EFA	essential fatty acid
EFM	electronic fetal monitoring
EFW	estimated fetal weight
EPIS	episiotomy
FAD	fetal activity diary
FAS	fetal alcohol syndrome
FBS	fetal blood sample; fasting blood sugar
FBM	fetal breathing movements
FHR	fetal heart rate
FHT	fetal heart tones
FM	fetal movement
FMD	fetal movement diary
FMR	fetal movement record
FPG	fasting plasma glucose
GDM	gestational diabetes mellitus
GI	gastrointestinal
GRAV	gravida
GTT	glucose tolerance test
GYN	gynecology
HCG	human chorionic gonadotrophin
HEENT	head, ears, eyes, nose, throat
HIV	human immunodeficiency virus
IDDM	insulin-dependent diabetes mellitus
IGT	impaired glucose tolerance
ITP	idiopathis thrombocytopenic purpura
IUFD	intrauterine fetal demise
IUGR	intrauterine growth retardation
IV	intravenous
JCAHO	Joint Commission for the Accreditation of Healthcare Organizations
L/S ratio	lecithin/sphingomyelin ratio
MAP	mean arterial pressure
NIDDM	non–insulin-dependent diabetes mellitus
NPO	nulla per os
NSCT	nipple stimulation challenge test
NST	non-stress test
OB	obstetric

OCT	oxytocin challenge test
PIH	pregancy-induced hypertension
PO	per os (by mouth)
PROM	premature rupture of membranes
RBC	red blood cell
RDS	Respiratory distress syndrome
RMA	right mentoanterior
ROA	right occiput anterior
ROM	rupture of membranes
ROP	right occiput posterior
ROP	retinopathy of prematurity
ROT	right occiput transverse
RMP	right mentoposterior
RMT	right mentotransverse
RSA	right sacroanterior
RSP	right sacroposterior
SFD	small for dates
SGA	small for gestational age
SIDS	sudden infant death syndrome
SOAP	subjective data, objective data, analysis, plan
SOB	short of breath
SROM	spontaneous rupture of the membranes
STD	sexually transmitted disease
TORCH	toxoplasmosis, other (viruses) rubella, cytomegalovirus, herpes virus type 2
TPN	total parenteral nutrition
TSS	toxic shock syndrome
U/A	urinalysis
UAC	umbilical artery catheter
UC	uterine contraction
UPI	uteroplacental insufficiency
UTI	urinary tract infection
VBAC	vaginal birth after cesarean
WBC	white blood cell
WIC	supplemental food program for woman, infants, and children
WNL	within normal limits

Glossary

abortion	loss of pregnancy before the fetus is viable outside the uterus; miscarriage, or elective termination
abruptio placentae	partial or total premature separation of a normally implanted placenta
acceleration	increase in the baseline fetal heart
acme	peak; time of greatest intensity (of a uterine contraction)
acrocyanosis	cyanosis of the extremities
afterbirth	placenta and membranes expelled or "delivered" after the infant; referred to as the third stage of labor
afterbirth pains	cramplike pains due to contractions of the uterus after childbirth
albinism	a congenital absence of normal skin pigmentation
albuminuria	readily detectable amounts of albumin in the urine
amenorrhea	suppression or absence of menstruation
amniocentesis	removal of amniotic fluid by insertion of needle into the amniotic sac (amniotic fluid is used to assess health and maturity status of fetus)
amnion	the inner of the two uterine membranes that form the sac containing the fetus and the amniotic fluid
amniotic fluid	the fluid surrounding the fetus in utero
amnionitis	infection within the amniotic fluid
amniotomy	the artificial rupturing of the amniotic sac
analgesic	drug that relieves pain
anencephaly	congenital deformity in which the cerebrum, cerebellum, and flat bones of the skull are absent
anesthesia	partial or complete loss of sensation with or without loss of consciousness; excess amount of carbon dioxide in the body
anomaly	a malformation; an organ or structure
anoxia	deficiency of oxygen
antepartum	time between conception and the onset of labor
anterior	pertaining to the front
Apgar score	a scoring system used to evaluate newborns at 1 minute and 5 minutes after delivery. The total score is derived by assessing five signs: heart rate, respiratory effort, muscle tone, reflex irritability, and color
apnea	a condition that occurs when respirations cease for more than 20 seconds, with cyanosis
areola	darker pigmented skin surrounding the nipple of the breast
Bartholin's glands	two small mucus glands on each side of the vaginal orifice that secrete small amounts of mucus during intercourse

bilirubin	orange or yellowish pigment in bile; a breakdown product of red blood cells that is carried by the blood to the liver, where it is excreted in the bile and in the stools
brown adipose tissue	fat deposits in neonates that provide greater heat protection
caudal block	regional anesthesia used in childbirth, given through the spinal canal
cephalhematoma	subcutaneous swelling found on the head of an infant several days after delivery
cephalic	referring to the head
cervical dilation	the cervical os and the cervical canal widen from less than 1 centimeter to approximately 10 centimeter
chloasma	brownish pigmentation over the bridge of the nose
chorion	one of the two uterine membranes closest to the intrauterine wall
Leopold's maneuvers	series of four maneuvers designed to allow the examiner to determine fetal presentation and position
mastitis	inflammation of the breast
neonatal mortality rate	number of deaths of infants in the first 28 days of life per 1,000 live births
neonate	infant from birth through the first 28 days of life
neonatology	the specialty that focuses on the management of high-risk conditions of the newborn
omphalitis	infection of the umbilicus
omphalocele	congential herniation of abdominal contents into the base of the umbilicus
outlet dystocia	inadequate pelvic size, causing the fetal head to be pushed backward toward the coccyx, making delivery of head difficult
ovum	female reproductive cell; egg
oxygen toxicity	serious, sometimes irreversible damage to pulmonary capillary endothelium associated with excessive levels of oxygen therapy
oxytocics	drugs that stimulate uterine contractions
oxytocin	hormone normally produced by the posterior pituitary, responsible for stimulation of uterine contractions and the release of milk into the lactiferous ducts
oxytocin challenge test (OCT)	also called the contraction stress test (CCST), the test evaluates the circulatory and respiratory status of the fetoplacental unit
palpation	use of fingers or hands to manually perform assessment
perforation of the uterus	a hole made in the uterus
perineum	the area of tissue between the anus and vagina in the female
periodic breathing	sporadic episodes of apnea, not associated with cyanosis, lasting about 10 seconds
persistent pulmonary hypertension	a neonatal syndrome secondary to pulmonary hypertension; seen in preterm but more frequently in full-term and postmature infants
phenylketonuria (PKU)	a recessive hereditary metabolic error that causes the buildup of phenylalanine, leading to mental retardation, brain damage, light pigmentation and other growth deformities. It is treated with a low-phenylalanine diet
phlebitis	inflammation of a vein

phototherapy	treatment of newborn jaundice by exposure to natural or special artificial light
physiologic jaundice	harmless condition caused by the normal reduction of red blood cells, occurs usually between the second and fifth day after birth, peaking on the fifth to seventh day, and disappearing between the seventh and tenth day.
placenta previa	improper implantation of the placenta on the lower uterine segment. Classification of type is based on closeness to the cervical os: total—completely covers the os; partial—covers a portion of the os; marginal—in close proximity to the os
preterm infant	any infant born before 37 weeks' gestation
preterm labor	labor beginning before the 37th week of gestation
primipara	a woman who has given birth to her first child
postmature infant	a newborn that is overly developed or that is more than 42 weeks' gestation
postnatal	occurring after birth
precipitous delivery	unduly rapid progression of labor
preeclampsia	toxemia of pregnancy; characterized by hypertension, albuminuria, and edema
pregnancy-induced hypertension (PIH)	a hypertensive disorder including preeclampsia and eclampsia as conditions; identified by the three cardinal signs: hypertension, edema, and proteinuria
prolapsed cord	umbilical cord that becomes compressed in the vagina before the fetus is delivered, resulting in emergency situation for the fetus
prolonged labor	labor lasting more than 24 hours
puerperium	the period after completion of the third stage of labor until involution of the uterus is complete at about 6 weeks
quickening	the first fetal movements felt by the pregnant woman, usually between 16 and 18 weeks' gestation
rales	an abnormal respiratory sound caused by air passing through fluid in the alveoli and bronchioles
regional anesthesia	injection of local anesthetic
rhonchi	coarse, abnormal auscultatory sounds
saddle block anesthesia	sensory and motor anesthesia of the buttocks, perineum, and inner aspects of the thighs, produced by spinal or intrathecal injection
show	a pinkish mucous discharge from the vagina that may occur a few hours to a few days before the onset of labor
spina bifida occulta	a defect in the vertebrae of the spinal column without protrusion of neural components
subinvolution	failure of a part to return to its normal size
surfactant	a surface-active mixture of secreted lipoproteins caused by *Candida albicans*, in the alveoli and air passages; it reduces surface tension of pulmonary fluids and contributes to the elasticity of lung tissue
tachycardia	abnormally rapid heart rate
tachypnea	excessively rapid respirations
term infant	a liveborn infant at 38 to 42 weeks' gestation
thromboembolus	thrombotic material or clot within the vein
tocodynamometer	external device that can be used to estimate uterine contraction pressures during labor

umbilical cord	the structure connecting the placenta to the umbilicus of the fetus through which the fetus receives nutrition and eliminates wastes
urinary meatus	external opening of the urethra
uterus	the hollow muscular organ in which the fertilized egg is implanted and in which the developing fetus is nourished until birth
vagina	the musculomembranous tube located between the external genitals and the uterus
varicose veins	permanently distended veins
vasectomy	surgical removal of a portion of the vas deferens

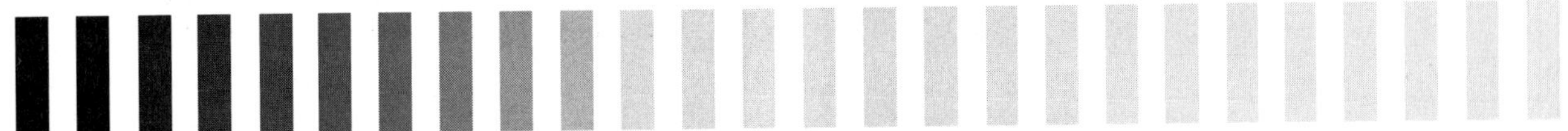

Index

Page numbers followed by *t* indicate tables; those followed by *b* indicate boxes.